Featured on the cover: The silhouette was adopted from a photo of Pearlina, a Liberian girl who was admitted to an ebola treatment unit for observation and later released. She never had Ebola. The photo was taken by M. Holden Warren for More Than Me, a local organization http://www.morethanme.org/blog/meet-pearlina-2/. Used with permission. Sources of the other photos from left to right are: An ebola medic (www.delcf.org), a nurse (More Than Me), Mercy washing (http://instagram.com/p/sanwr_DsF1, More Than Me) and Isata Konneh, an ebola survivor featured on UNICEF's blog (http://blogs.unicef.org/2014/08/07/ebola-in-sierra-leone-the-joy-of-survivors).

Ebola
Real Voices, Hard Facts.
By Marc Maxmeister
Copywrite 2014
Table of Contents

Introduction

Ebola is one of the greatest threats modern society has ever faced, but not for the reasons you might have heard. It compels good people to do great things and not-so-good people to do horrible things.

I wrote this book because I was appalled by all the misinformation. I first considered writing it in August of 2014 when I scanned the kindle ebook store and found an new book on Ebola written for the "preppers" community. The "preppers"[1] are a fringe group that plans for the eventual breakdown of the social fabric - the canned food and shotgun stockpiling crowd. Not only was the tone of this book alarmist, the information about the disease was just plain wrong. Nevertheless, by October it had over 50 five-star reviews and hundreds (perhaps thousands) of copies sold. There are hundreds of full-time misinformers out there - they want your money, not your well-being. And so I decided to do something about it.

Given that I happened to be a scientist and I had been reading the actual peer-reviewed journal articles on Ebola, its projections, and how to contain it, I felt I needed to digest them for a general audience. But I also wanted to infuse these facts with as much first-hand perspective as I could, from the people who are battling Ebola in West Africa. I've spent years living in various parts of Africa, running a giant storytelling project with a nonprofit called GlobalGiving. My work has been a search for ways to let citizens speak for themselves about what they want and who is or is not giving it to them. Now, more than ever, someone needed to project their voices out above the noise.

Ebola is a lot like corruption and poverty in one respect - it can affect everyone in one society and be ignored in another until its effects boil over. But when the problem boils over, the people who've ignored the root cause too often go on ignoring the people who really understand it. Their stories are not collected and never heard. This is my attempt to give the people of Liberia and Sierra Leone their chance to tell the story.

It is more than simply believing they "deserve a voice." Their local knowledge is our best asset in the fight to contain this global epidemic. We will need to learn from people who have first-hand knowledge of the disease if we want to stand a chance of stopping it. The conventional playbook - which calls for us to fly doctors in and put up quarantines - is not working, as you will see. What will ultimately work is going to be different from what's worked before.

As of December, 2014 the Ebola epidemic had not been contained. Every person that contracts the disease still infects two more on average. This is low compared to other airborne diseases like the measles, but that number needs to be less than one in order for the disease to stop spreading. 37 percent of everyone who has ever contracted Ebola since its discovery in 1976 got it in the last two weeks alone. That statement was true when I wrote it in October of 2014, but it was also true in September, and in August before that. It is a good example of how newspapers churn out alarm bell headlines that are merely math. If you are facing exponential growth of a virus in a population, about a third of all new cases will have occurred in the last X days, where X is whatever the incubation time is. For Ebola, X is two weeks. If one person infects two more, the number affected should double every two weeks. This is the definition of "not contained" but there is something you can do about it. You can remain calm, educate yourself on the hard facts, and understand why the outbreak got so bad. For example, when the outbreak first took hold in Liberia, there were only eight ambulances and 200 hospital beds for four million people. It also took months for a string of mysterious deaths to be recognized as Ebola. Europe and America have far greater capacity to deal with outbreaks, and we won't experience an epidemic unless panicky people bring down the system with counterproductive behavior.

The way that news media and a mostly American group of scare-bloggers talked about Ebola preyed on the ignorance of the American people. Science education in America failed on a civic level - most citizens don't know how science works and don't trust "the facts." We care more about "whose facts" we should believe. When nine out of ten people get their news from a questionable source and cannot tell the difference between truth from the CDC and "truth" from disasterresponseteamofamerica.wordpress.com, public health problems become threats to society itself. Many of the people reading these disreputable blogs already distrust their government, and that distrust creates a self-fulfilling prophecy whereby the government cannot do its job and protect the people. Democratic governments rely on the people to voluntarily cooperate with laws such as quarantines and turn dictatorial when the people resist. This is exactly what happened with the West Point quarantine in Liberia's capitol, Monrovia, as you will learn. The same chaos would play out on a larger scale if we imposed a travel ban on whole countries, or if citizens ignored the requests of governments.

It is hard to introduce a book meant to counteract the alarmist voices without myself sounding alarmist. The threat of Ebola is real, but if you live in America your risk of getting Ebola is close to zero. The real threat is the way that we all change when presented with an existential threat like Ebola. Do we become heroes, like many of the people I will introduce here, or do we resort to profiteering, spreading conspiracy theories, and vomiting our racially -motivated distrust of the "other" into the gutters of the Internet? Most of us don't know what kind of person we really are until a crisis forces us to choose. Would you share what little you had if you were trapped inside a quarantine and food was running out? Would you smuggle your grandmother or daughter through a tunnel to see a doctor and save a life? Or would you obey the rules and contain the threat for the good of the many? Would you still do it if you knew your government was doing nothing to save your life?

If you are holding an ebook reader, you and I live a red carpet existence. Conquering our own fear is our greatest challenge. A crisis like Ebola forces us to stand on a razor's edge and examine both sides. Each bad decision raises the stakes on the next decision. Leaders that chose the simpler path of quarantine found it quickly backfire. Had they not reconsidered, we would be looking at many more untraceable Ebola cases turning up in unexpected places now. But convincing the people to go along with the tougher decision - even if it is the right one - brings its own challenge. This book is about the tough decisions and the solutions. By understanding what has already happened, I hope we may all understand the tough choices. After all, what we decide determines whether we rise above or slip into evil.

---

[1] http://www.motherjones.com/politics/2012/11/preppers-survivalist-doomsday-obama

1: Where did this West African Ebola outbreak come from?

The first case came in December of 2013 in the town of Gueckedou, Guinea[1]. This town is 5 miles from the intersection of three countries - Guinea, Sierra Leone, and Liberia. A two year old boy died with flu-like symptoms and a week later his mother died with a confirmed case of Ebola. Pretty soon the boy's sister and grandmother fell ill, followed by the village midwife.

Ebola has many symptoms that are indistinguishable from the flu. The original charts on these patients lists their symptoms as fever, diarrhea, and vomiting for most of the patients, but a few had hemorrhaging and spontaneous abortions. There was one major clue too minor to make it into doctors' charts: some patients had hiccups, a benign side-effect of Ebola, something not found with similar diseases like cholera and malaria. Notes about hiccups found its way through email chains to an expert at MSF that ordered them tested for Ebola.[2] Ebola had never been seen in West Africa before, so it was an odd request. The PCR tests confirmed the Zaire Ebola virus (EBOV) was present in their blood,[3] and in March of 2013 this cluster of mysterious deaths was recognized by doctors to be Ebola.

From December to May, many funerals were held in a region spanning three countries. In Liberia and Sierra Leone, the custom when someone dies is for the family to wash the body. Then mourners lay their hands on the body, wiping, massaging, kissing and embracing it as a sign of deep respect. These are sacred burial rituals and no other common diseases in West Africa - malaria, aids - are spread by touching the body after death, so it was not immediately recognized as a risk. Ebola is the opposite of the flu because a carrier is not contagious early on, and shows no sign of the virus in saliva (sneezing) and mucus (coughing) until a fever appears. But once the patient starts to hemorrhage, he is very contagious, and becomes *most contagious* after death.

As more people died of the mystery disease, sick people traveled farther in search of healers. A renown healer lived about 80 miles away from Gueckedou in the diamond-mining town of

Kiodu, Eastern Sierra Leone. She would treat patients with herbal remedies and by laying her hands on them. She too contracted Ebola, fell ill, and died. They held a massive funeral in May where 14 women touched her body as many as 365 people are believed to have died as a result[4,5].

By May health authorities had caught on and quickly tried to bring an end to the practice of mourners touching the deceased, but the outbreak had already grown beyond the capacity of the local healthcare system. Liberia had an estimated 8 ambulances and 200 hospital beds for over 4 million people, with similar estimates in Sierra Leone and Guinea.

By mid-June, an explosive outbreak was clearly under way in nearby Kailahun. The government hospital was overwhelmed. Twelve nurses were quickly infected and died, forcing authorities to close and quarantine the hospital. Soon after the international NGO Doctors Without Borders had moved in to help. One local account[6]:

> A walk through the steamy streets of Kailahun is an unexpectedly uplifting experience, given that almost everyone knows someone who has died of Ebola. Children play noisily to a soundtrack of fire finches, egrets and emerald cuckoos, chasing old tyres in the iron-rich red mud, while adults throng the streets exchanging money, black-market petrol and laughter. But the atmosphere changes a short walk uphill at the specialist Ebola treatment centre run by global aid charity Doctors without Borders, known by its French acronym MSF. Here, there is little joy, nor reason to laugh — only death and suffering.

> The centre runs like a military camp, everyone following procedure to the letter, every patient and health worker divided by location and clothing according to their risk status. Patients brought to the centre leave with certificates confirming their recovery, or in heavily disinfected body bags. Most of her patients suffer severe diarrhoea, vomiting and agonising pain as their organs break down, which is eased by morphine and

tramadol. "I'm feeling the pain. I have pain in my joints, which they are treating," she tells AFP from behind two plastic fences that create a protective buffer zone a few feet wide. "The worst pain I feel though is whenever I see the other children here running around, sick with Ebola."

Leaving town, a black-topped highway bordered by palm trees and flat, endless savannah eventually gives way to a treacherous mud track lined by crocodile-infested swampland, dense forests. At a checkpoint police bark questions at each traveler, demanding proof of accreditation to go further. At three of the posts, people are made to wash their hands in chlorine and have their temperatures taken.

"We are so sad because our brothers and sisters are dying, so many of them," a police guard explains, at a post on the border between Kenema and Kailahun districts.

The recent history of this part of the world provides more context as to why it took nearly six months for an Ebola outbreak to be recognized here. Both Sierra Leone and Liberia fell into a generation-long civil war at the end of the cold war. With the sudden loss of American and Soviet aid to local dictators, diamonds became the new prize, and warlords popped up to claim those prizes. This foreign peacemaker's account describes the situation nearly 20 years later:[7]

You could write the story of the war through the daily images of life in Kono, Sierra Leone: The burned down houses and structures that are now being occupied by families-despite the lack of covering overhead; The devastated infrastructure; The mines-small and large-we pass daily to get from our guest house to the heart of town everyday. It is hard to imagine the violence and suffering that happened on these lands.

As we were passing one of the many burned houses today, I saw corn growing up through the blackened cement structure that remains a memorial of the war-a constant reminder to the people here. There is life growing out of the devastation. In our encounters at the market, in the friendships we are making at the guest house, and in our relationships with those we are interviewing and meeting with, I am constantly astounded by their resiliency and love.

1000 child soldiers were reintegrated into Kono. Reconciliation and healing is still taking place, but the very fact that people have found ways to live together-to move beyond means of violence in what is still a very contentious area is an incredible example of the power of the human spirit.

Kono was the heart of the disputed diamond-mining district; now it is near the epicenter of the Ebola epidemic. The region was not functionally integrated into any national government, leaving it particularly susceptible to Ebola. Nobody was watching.

So where did this outbreak come from? While scientists speculate about bats or tainted bush meat as the source, the ethnographer would say that lawlessness created it and a culture of corruption and elitism enabled it to escape early quarantines. More on that story is to come.

---

[1] New England Journal of Medicine http://www.nejm.org/doi/full/10.1056/NEJMoa1404505#t=article

[2] http://nymag.com/scienceofus/2014/09/how-hiccups-helped-doctors-identify-ebola.html

[3] http://currents.plos.org/outbreaks/article/phylogenetic-analysis-of-guinea-2014-ebov-ebolavirus-outbreak-2/

[4] http://www.nytimes.com/2014/08/29/health/ebola-outbreak-in-sierra-leone-is-tied-to-one-funeral.html?_r=0

[5] http://www.who.int/csr/disease/ebola/ebola-6-months/sierra-leone/en/

[6] http://reliefweb.int/report/sierra-leone/suffering-and-song-sierra-leones-ebola-hot-zone

[7] http://www.catalystforpeace.org/voicetovision/blog/first-day-in-kono-sierra-leone/

2: Will the outbreak be contained?

Aha! That's the big question. First I need to cover the evidence that epidemiologists use when predicting whether Ebola is spreading at a faster or slower rate. From what we have learned since 1976, Ebola kills most of the people who contract it, but each infected person doesn't spread it to that many more people. The numbers that seem stable for this 2014 epidemic are 2 and 70. For every person who gets Ebola, two other people will contract it from him within the next two-to-three weeks, and 70 percent of those people will die. The 30 percent that survive will have Ebola antibodies in their blood and be effectively immune to the disease. This is really important for modeling. It means Ebola will not kill us all, no matter what you've heard. It won't even kill off millions of people, because it is relatively hard to catch and somewhat treatable in a hospital. Even though 70 percent die, that number is higher (85 percent) if the patient is not receiving any treatment, and a little lower (50 to 60 percent) if they are receiving the best available treatment.

So how is a patient treated? Once a person has been diagnosed, we can provide them with intravenous (IV) fluids to counteract the most serious effect of the disease - the rapid dehydration. In the later stages of the disease, small blood clots form in vessels throughout the body, and through a different mechanism, Ebola causes internal bleeding. This combination of effects causes most organs to fail unless a person's fluid and electrolyte balance is maintained. That is the "hemorrhagic fever" you may have heard about in the news[1]. Internal hemorrhaging can sometimes cause purple spots on the skin but usually does not. Hospitalization does increase the survival rate[2] by reducing internal bleeding.

The prediction models for how many people are likely to get Ebola in the near future have to fit real numbers to get realistic predictions. One recent model that I like because it is very transparent about its assumptions and corrections for misinformation assumes that as of August 2014, there were 2.5 times more people with Ebola than the official numbers reported[3].

This discrepancy started when the number of cases exceeded the number of hospital beds, so families stopped bringing their people in for treatment. The paper also models out the likely success rate of home treatment and isolation (with people educating families on what precautions to take) over trying to cram everyone into hospitals or failing to do proper education. It finds that home isolation is almost as good as a hospital quarantine in West Africa at stopping the spread of the disease, albeit with lower survival rates of Ebola patients outside of hospitals.

One encouraging real life example of home isolation and treatment comes from Fatu Kekula[4]:

> Fatu was in her final year of nursing school in Liberia when her whole family fell victim to Ebola. You would think that given her profession, she could get them special treatment in a hospital, but the system was overloaded. Fatu escorted her father hours away to Monrovia, over difficult roads. Three hospitals turned them away because they were full. So she took him back to smaller hospital in Kakata. They said he had typhoid fever, which was wrong. Fatu took him home, where he infected three other family members: Fatu's mother, sister, and their 14-year-old cousin.

> 22-year-old Fatu nursed her entire family through Ebola out of necessity. She constructed a makeshift isolation ward in an unfinished room in their home. She improvised her own equipment, patching together a HAZMAT suit from trash bags as her protective gear. She put on a rubber raincoat, then put trash bags over her socks and tied them in a knot over her calves. She stuffed them into thick rubber boots, then wore more trash bags over her boots. She wrapped her hair in a pair of stockings and over that a trash bag. She wore rubber gloves and a face mask.

> Despite the 100-degree weather, Fatu followed a strict suiting-up regimen every day, several times a day, for about two weeks.

All of these items were available in the local market, but she understood the discipline it required to use them effectively, due to her prior nursing training. She never cut corners.

She fed them and cleaned them on a regular schedule. She gave them medications to treat the symptoms and improvised an IV fluid drip for each member of her family. She monitored their vital signs and minimized the damage from the hemorrhagic fever during the worse of it. Three out of her four patients survived. That's a 25% death rate - considerably better than the 70 percent death rate for Ebola patients in the hospitals there. Ingenuity helped Fatu save her family, and she never caught Ebola herself. In the same month, more than 300 health care workers became infected with Ebola because they did not follow the same precautions meticulously.

While operating her one-woman Ebola hospital for two weeks, Fatu consulted with their family doctor, who would talk to her on the phone, but wouldn't come to the house. She gave them medicines she obtained from the local clinic and fluids through intravenous lines that she started.

At times, her patients' blood pressure plummeted so low she feared they would die.

"I cried many times," she said. "I said 'God, you want to tell me I'm going to lose my entire family?' "

But her father, mother, and sister rallied and were well on their way to recovery when space became available at a local hospital nearly two-weeks later. Her cousin Alfred never recovered, though, and passed away at the hospital the next day.

"I'm very, very proud," her father said. "She saved my life through the almighty God."

Now he's working to find a scholarship for Fatu so she can finish her final year of nursing school. He has no doubt his daughter will go on to save many more people during her life.

International aid workers who later heard about Fatu's "trash bag method" began teaching it to other West Africans who couldn't get into hospitals and don't have protective gear of their own. It became apparent that relying on the existing healthcare system to treat every Ebola patient was unsustainable as the scale of the outbreak grew. By August 2014 practically every hospital bed in Liberia was serving an Ebola victim, leaving none to treat other diseases like malaria, aids, and tuberculosis. The pragmatic approach was to turn homes into clinics and train people to avoid spreading Ebola once it infected a home. There is no exact way to predict how effective this will be, because it depends less on how many people are "taught" and more on how well people actually understand how this disease spreads. However, it is far more likely to work when the few hundred hospital beds in Liberia are overrun by the tens of thousands of infected people than any other approach. And people have an amazing capacity to learn when their lives are on the line.

"Essentially this is a tale of how communities are doing things for themselves," a UNICEF spokesperson said. "Our approach is to listen and work with communities and help them do the best they can with what they have." That approach is the most conservative way to ensure success when facing a complex problem. In November Doctors Without Borders (MSF) distributed hundreds of thousands of home Ebola kits to citizens with gloves and disinfectant spray in them, preparing for the inevitable.

So back to the big question, can Ebola be contained? The best answer is "It depends."

IF the population at risk can be re-educated on how to avoid spreading the disease when exposed, and

IF the required change in one's behavior is not too difficult to sustain for months at a time, and

IF male Ebola survivors can be coaxed into avoiding sex for months afterwards, and

IF politicians avoid the temptation to impose a simplistic tactic to a complex problem, it can be contained.

Note that there a lot of IFs in my answer. It depends on behavior change, on leaders and survivors being capable of unpopular long-term thinking, and on replacing old unsafe behaviors with safer ones that are not draconian. For example, expecting every citizen in West Africa to wear hazmat suits in 100+ degree weather is draconian and unrealistic, as is the suggestion that they "just stop touching each other." It is far simpler to replace common social triggers with safer alternatives. One example of a behavior swap was to popularize elbow bumping instead of handshaking:[5]

From Mila Rosenthal, UNDP worker:

Am I scared for myself being here, in the countries where people are suffering an outbreak of a nightmare? Honestly, not much. Yes, I know Ebola is serious, but I know how it's transmitted.

Let me describe one experience on a high-level UN delegation on Ebola: you are met at the airport in Guinea, the capital of Conakry. At the entrance to the hotel, there is a barrel of bleach-laced water for disinfectant, and you wash your hands in it. A guard checks your temperature with a thermometer that doesn't touch the skin. You are not feverish, so you go in.

At the entrance to UN offices and government offices, you wash your hands in decontaminant again and get your temperature checked again. There are bottles of hand sanitizer on every table and they are regularly passed around like gum, and everyone takes a squirt. You get briefed on the situation. You plan how you can improve UNDP's work to prevent further contagion and support everyone who is even poorer and worse off because Ebola has derailed trade and jobs and food and schools. When you visit programmes and meet staff and volunteers working in the communities, they are on the frontlines of pushing the prevention message and living it too. You wash your hands in bleach again. You get your temperature checked again.

This is pretty low risk stuff from a personal health point of view, I must say. Everyone smells like chlorine and bleach and hand sanitizer. No one has a fever, that's for sure.

And no one shakes hands.

This no-hand-shaking is destabilizing to an American me, for whom extending one's hand in introductory greeting is a deeply ingrained instinct. I know from working in West Africa that it is equally ingrained here—a handshake and a friendly pat on the shoulder is a common way to start even the slightest encounter. It was a common way. Now, no.

The mix of foreigners and Guineans, Sierra Leoneans, and Liberians I've met on this trip take a variety of different approaches to the no-touching problem. One is the **Ebola elbow bump**. This is what it sounds like: two people face each other and extend their opposite cocked elbows up to each other. A variation is the Ebola fist bump, which does the same thing at waist level with the outside of a closed fist. The Cuban epidemiologist we met in Sierra Leone eschewed the bumps, saying all contact could be risky: instead, he put his hand over his heart and bobbed his head forward in a courtly bow. In one government office, I watched the Foreign Minister walk down the hall and bump elbows with the rest of the Cabinet as he passed.

When the disease is so devastating, it may seem like a silly diversion to be troubled that I can't shake a guy's hand. But I can't really tame my body from the habit of doing it. My right hand thrusts itself out involuntarily in meeting after meeting. My hosts glance down at the offending paw with bemusement or dismissal. Finally, as the days go on, the inadvertent hand thrust is reduced to a repressed spasm, and then to a mere twitch. My hand remembers the instinct, my brain smothers it.

This simple behavior change is about the biggest adjustment that whole populations can realistically expect to absorb in under two-weeks. You contact other people and the residue left behind from other people dozens of times every day. And getting male survivors to abstain for nearly three months is harder still.

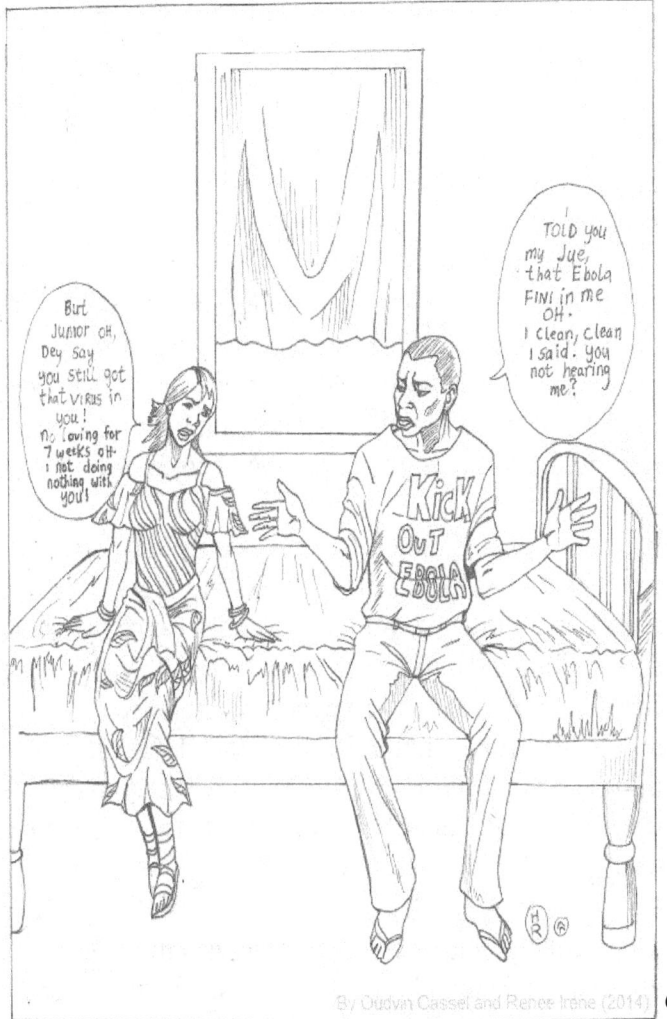

By Oydvin Cassel and Renee Irene (2014) 6

That is why the real risk in 2015 is that Ebola, once contained, becomes a persistent sexually-transmitted disease. The longest lasting viral reservoir in humans is semen.

Yet even harder than avoiding all contact with the human race and enforcing moratoriums on sex **is getting politicians to think long-term**. On Nov 3, 2014 the Australian minister for immigration suspended immigration from Ebola affected regions, including humanitarian travelers. "Australia is canceling or refusing visas for people from Ebola-affected nations," he said.[7]

Closing the border would actually increase the likelihood of Ebola getting into the country undetected. Right now we know the exact identity and number of people coming in from Liberia to the US or Australia, and we know when they were last healthy (through airport temperature checks). All US flights from affected countries now come into five airports with specialized staff prepared to deal with Ebola. We're dealing with the problem from a regulatory mindset. The alternative is a prohibition mindset that would achieve the desired result about as well as alcohol prohibition worked in the US in the 1920s and 1930s. The real threat here are self-serving and ideological politicians creating health policies with willful ignorance of how people will react to their policies.

CDC director Thomas Freiden said, "The only way we're going to get to zero risk is by stopping the outbreak at the source. Even if we tried to close the border, it wouldn't work. Because by isolating these countries, it'll make it harder to help them; it'll spread more there, and we'd be more likely to be exposed here."[8] A spokesperson for Doctors Without Borders added, "Lockdowns and quarantines do not help control Ebola as they end up driving people underground and jeopardizing the trust between people and health providers."[9]

Yet there remains a large disconnect between realistic strategies that work and the simplistic sound byte strategies that politicians lean on for votes. A recent poll in the US conservative newspaper *The Washington Times* showed a startlingly high percentage of its readers wanted America to close its borders. To the question, "Should the U.S. close its borders to flights from West Africa to contain the Ebola outbreak?" 93 percent said yes.[10]

And naturally, conservative politicians are parroting what their conservative constituents want to hear. Senator Ted Cruz (R) of Texas said:

Common sense dictates that we should impose a travel ban on commercial airline flights from nations afflicted by Ebola. There's no reason to allow ongoing commercial air traffic out of those countries. Health care personnel can be brought in on military C-130 flights instead. The risks of epidemic are far too large for us to allow unimpeded commercial flights.[11]

Texas governor Rick Perry:

Air travel is how this disease crosses borders. I believe it is the right policy to ban air travel from countries that have been hit hardest by the Ebola outbreak.[12]

Previously he had been against a ban, but changed his mind. Changing one's policies about a travel ban depending on public opinion is a tactic that both Republicans and Democrats have done. In North Carolina Democratic Senator Kay Hagan opposed a ban until she changed her mind too, weeks before an election:

I have said for weeks that travel restrictions should be one part of a broad strategy to prevent Ebola from spreading in the U.S. and fighting it in Africa. I am calling on the Administration to temporarily ban the travel of non-U.S. citizens from the affected countries in West Africa. Although stopping the spread of this virus overseas will require a large, coordinated effort with the international community, a temporary travel ban is a prudent step the President can take to protect the American people, and I believe he should do so immediately.

These politicians are thinking about the next election and not about a disease on an exponential trajectory. More importantly, they're in denial of the complex system we must deal with. Ebola is carried by people, and people will always find a way through a closed border if they really want to. Contact spreads the disease in the medical sense, but human ingenuity spreads the disease in the psychosocial sense. And whenever a few people try to impose their will on the masses, the masses find a way to squirm out from under the heavy hand. It was an ironic coincidence that opposite the *NY Times* article about Australia closing its borders was a curiosity about most popular highlighted quote in the kindle copy of *Lord of the Rings*:

> The wide world is all about you: you can fence yourselves in, but you cannot for ever fence it out.

Mila's recent essay shows the more pragmatic way that people in the epicenter of this epidemic are dealing with it, and America would be wise to adopt the same approach.

[1] http://en.wikipedia.org/wiki/Viral_hemorrhagic_fever

[2] I am still looking for a reference as to how much. The fact that nobody publishes this means it is probably only 10 or 20 percent lower. Untreat Ebola epidemics in the 1970s had a greater than 90 percent death rate in Zaire (now DRC), but under constant supervision with the best medical care, as many as 70 percent survive.

[3] http://www.cdc.gov/mmwr/pdf/other/su6303.pdf

[4] http://www.cnn.com/2014/09/25/health/ebola-fatu-family/

[5] http://www.undp.org/content/undp/en/home/blog/2014/10/17/Hands-free-diplomacy-on-Ebola/

[6] http://cassellandirene.tumblr.com/post/101860815742/ebola-style-life-in-lib-sign-of-the-times-one

[7] http://op-talk.blogs.nytimes.com/2014/11/07/australias-little-guantanamos/

[8] http://cnsnews.com/news/article/susan-jones/cdc-chief-even-if-we-tried-close-border-it-wouldnt-work

[9] http://in.reuters.com/article/2014/09/06/us-health-ebola-idINKBN0H10ID20140906

[10] http://www.washingtontimes.com/polls/2014/oct/3/should-us-close-its-borders-flights-west-africa-co/#ixzz3IaDn9xMq

[11] http://dailycaller.com/2014/10/15/ted-cruz-says-common-sense-dictates-an-ebola-travel-ban/

[12] http://hotair.com/archives/2014/10/17/quotes-of-the-day-1885/

3: Why not just find a cure or develop a vaccine for Ebola to stop its spread?

In versions of this story that must fit inside of two hours on a movie screen, the cliché ending is that a scientist develops a cure in the eleventh hour and distributes said cure to all the people in the world (off screen, because that's utter fantasy), followed by cheers and accolades for heroism. In reality, our first major vaccine - Jonas Salk's polio vaccine in 1952 - is still being rolled out to the last few countries in 2014. And that vaccine was never patented[1] and thus distributed more widely more quickly than any other vaccine since. And while a vaccine for Ebola seems likely to become a reality some time in 2015 (three different vaccines will be tested), it is not the single most important component to stopping the epidemic in the immediate future.

I mentioned before that what matters most is behavior change and getting leaders to consider the consequences of their policies on a global level. A vaccine will help after it is tested and millions of doses are available, but the promise of a vaccine is dangerous. If people put their faith in a future vaccine or cure instead of changing their behavior now, they maintain bad behaviors that accelerate the spread of disease.

Vaccinating the world is a difficult logistical challenge that will require international trust and cooperation. Add to that the time and risk it takes to grow huge 1000-liter vats of the virus that is needed to mass produce the vaccine, and you can see why behavior change is the only immediate solution. In October 2014 the one vaccine that appears to work (ZMapp) was in short supply. Perhaps only a dozen doses existed, which explains why nobody was getting treated with ZMapp in Liberia. The most recent estimates from a leaked WHO document are that pharma giant GlaxoSmithKline[2] (GSK) could have 230,000 doses ready for testing in West Africa by April of 2015, but are only guaranteeing 24,000 doses by January of 2015[3]. Hitting the larger production target would require lowering safety guidelines from bio safety level 4 to level 2. The less secure facilities stand a real chance of infecting workers. This means that if the public demanded vaccines for everybody, there would be a real risk that the GSK biofactory in Belgium with dozens of 1000-liter vats of Ebola could be the epicenter of its own outbreak. Luckily, no government official has endorsed this idea. But history shows that if the public demands it, some will.

GSK's competitor NewLink has promised 12 million doses of their concoction by the same time, provided some government agency was willing to pay the up-front cost of producing them. Vaccines are an investment product, not a public good. No for-profit company will risk producing one without assurances that their investment will be recuperated, with interest. The board of NewLink met earlier in 2014 to consider mass-producing a vaccine, but shelved the idea because demand wasn't high enough (e.g. the body count was too small). In the CEO's own words[4]:

> At first, the board didn't see much commercial potential in it. But when the crisis began to evolve, everybody was: "Let's go, let's make this happen." There was no hesitancy once the crisis began.

- Charles Link Jr, in *Science*, October 31, 2014.

The reluctance to absorb the cost is natural, given the high risk of failure. None of these three remedies - ZMapp, GSK, or NewLink - have undergone large scale randomized control clinical trials (RCTs) and so there is no guarantee they will work most of the time for most of the people who take them. They show promise in a lab setting, and have worked with a handful of people who took them in the case of ZMapp, but most drug candidates do not make it through the FDA approval process. By the numbers since 1986[5], about 300 new drugs have been approved by the FDA from a pool of 5,400 candidates that were tested on humans in clinical trials. Over 50,000 distinct molecules started the process. Overall, 99.4 percent of new molecules failed to make it to market. Curing disease is a business, and the only way that any of these companies will guarantee an immediate supply of an untested drug is if the government absorbs all the costs up-front, which could be a $75 million dollar bill. For comparison, MSF built a dozen emergency hospitals and doubled the size of the healthcare system in West Africa in 2014 for less than this amount.

On the other hand, it seems likely that at least one of these will pass the test and make it to market. The science behind it is well-understood, and far less difficult than creating a vaccine for HIV. HIV attacks specific cells in the immune system that a vaccine would need intact to inoculate a person.

The more interesting debate is over new ways to test these drugs. Randomized Controlled Trials (RCTs) are the only standard design recognized by the FDA. In standard drug trials, neither the people receiving the drug nor the physicians prescribing the pill know whether they are giving the real pill or a sugar pill substitute (a placebo). A "double blind" design is needed because overwhelming empirical evidence shows that humans behave differently when they know they are in the treatment group or control group. If they believe they are in the treatment group, they get better and report fewer side-effects, even when they were given no drug. And conversely, people who believe they are in the control group sometimes show no improvement in the treatment group. This demonstrates that the mind has far more power to augment or suppress our natural disease resistance than science has yet been able to explain. The placebo effect is quite large - 35% of people consistently report it. There is even a biochemical basis for it in the case of pain. People with a specific variant of catechol-O-methyl-transferase, an enzyme that breaks down neurotransmitters (including the reward-related chemical dopamine), are far more likely to experience placebo pain relief or healing than the general population[6]. This makes it twice as hard to demonstrate that a drug works. The placebo effect also creates a secondary ethical problem. People who believe they are safe take more risks, and 70 percent of those in the control group are likely to die if exposed to Ebola.

The flip-side of the double blind design is that doctors treat patients differently if they know which patient is on the drug.

Perhaps they probe the control subjects less for mentions of side-effects to taking a sugar pill, or interview people in the treatment group more carefully. Another effective approach is a double blind study with a crossover design. This ensures that everybody get the treatment either for the first half or the second half of the experiment.

None of these approaches are ethical with an Ebola vaccine. No medic wants to go in and treat patients with a deadly disease if there is only a 50 percent chance the pill they just took will protect them, or a 100 percent chance they are unprotected 50 percent of the time with a crossover design. Moreover, vaccines are given once and last for years, so a crossover design is impossible.

The world's leading Ebola scientists debate these ethical dilemmas for hours in Geneva, Switzerland in October of 2014. Here were the various proposals, all alternatives to the standard RCT[7]:

"Going into this meeting, we were told the idea of a randomized controlled trial was not going to be acceptable," says Riplet Ballou, who heads the crash program to develop an Ebola vaccine at GlaxoSmithKline (GSK) in Rixensart, Belgium. In the efficacy tests for vaccines in West Africa, Ballou argued that half of the volunteers should randomly be assigned into a control arm—a group of people at risk of becoming infected who would not receive an experimental Ebola vaccine. Instead, they would serve as so-called active controls and be injected with other, approved vaccines, for instance against hepatitis B or pneumococcal disease. That would be the fastest way to know whether the Ebola vaccines work and can be deployed widely, Ballou said—and thus potentially save the most lives.

Representatives of Doctors Without Borders (MSF) were strongly opposed to giving trial participants anything other than an actual Ebola vaccine candidate.

A standard trial proves that a vaccine works by showing that more people in the control arm develop disease than those who got the actual vaccine, which would mean killing off dozens of people. They debated whether that was ethical, in a sense quantifying how many deaths would be worth preventing how many more deaths thereafter. Ballou presented illuminating estimates on the number of people expected to die in GSK's design. He assumed health care workers in Liberia would spend 10 percent of their time in direct contact with Ebola patients next year. Assuming the new vaccine worked 80 percent of the time, "researchers could be 'absolutely confident' about efficacy after 30 infections and within 3 months." 30 infections at a typical 70 percent fatality rate meant sacrificing 21 nurses and doctors in a vaccine trial. A less effective vaccine (60 percent efficacy) would yield an answer with 60 infections, 42 deaths.

While WHO experts and many other scientists considered this the best option, Doctors Without Borders refused to endorse this strategy.

The leading alternative is a design known as step-wedge, which essentially uses time to create a control group. In this design, researchers take advantage of the inescapable reality that large-scale trials can't give everyone the vaccine on the exact same date; they compare the rates of infection in people already vaccinated with those who have yet to receive the shots. Barney Graham, a virologist at NIAID in Bethesda, Maryland, who attended the meeting, says "people are more comfortable" with the step-wedge design, because everyone in such a study would get the Ebola vaccine.

The GSK vaccine only went into a human for the first time on September 2nd, 2014 in a phase I trial that will involve a few hundred volunteers not at risk of infection. If it is proven safe in healthy, unexposed people, 10,000 doses will be sent the three most affected countries in West Africa by January.

The meeting participants roundly agreed that it did not make sense to just give the experimental vaccines to health care workers on a so-called compassionate use basis and without an efficacy trial, as has happened with experimental

Ebola treatments such as ZMapp and TKM-Ebola; that strategy is simply too dangerous with a vaccine, which goes into healthy people.

"The attendees had a strong sense that there was no time to waste," especially after they were given an update on the situation in West Africa, Kieny says. "I was expecting more controversy." Looking back, "we basically said what people thought needed to be said but were afraid to say," Ballou says.

Jeremy Farrar, an infectious disease researcher who heads the Wellcome Trust research charity in London, thinks a randomized, controlled trial is ethical for the simple reason that no one really knows whether the vaccine will offer protection.

I believe there are other ways to prove a vaccine works without planning to sacrifice healthcare workers on the front lines, as has been suggested. While each of the scientists in that room was weighing the pros and cons of getting an answer to the question, "will this drug or that drug prevent the spread of Ebola?" they were also revealing to themselves what kind of person they wanted to be. How many lives are worth a cure? 21? And what if we have to run ten trials instead of just one? Are 210 people still worth it? Meanwhile, others were more willing to sacrifice rigor for the assurances that no one would - by design - be purposely put into a group that was expected to die at a higher rate. And yet this approach too ensures that more people outside of the experiment die as we await a vaccine.

Taking these positions to the extreme reveals much more about who were are, and how we value one life over another. If a disease were to threaten human extinction, advocates of the GSK trial would argue more vociferously for the blinding and control approach. Other advocates of using the standard approach were asking, "how can it be unethical to deny a drug to someone when we don't know if the drug works yet?" These are good philosophical questions in the hypothetical sense, but I'd prefer that we revisit the design instead of committing to save humanity by robbing us of that which makes us most human.[8] In our search for knowledge that can save lives, we should never be willing to sacrifice other innocent lives. That path always leads to even greater moral sacrifices.

We should also temper our haste by taking advantage of our natural immunity to disease, a cure that is beyond any commercial patenting. A survivor's immunity can be transferred to a sick person through a blood transfusion (if blood types are compatible), because survivors have Ebola antibodies and no longer have the virus in their blood. Several patients have been cured with another survivor's blood, even as far back as the original outbreak in 1976. The experimental serum ZMapp is actually an artificially grown concoction of antibodies based on the natural ones animals have grown to fight Ebola. So a vaccine is coming, but we will need to change community behaviors if we want to stop the epidemic altogether.

---

[1] http://www.forbes.com/sites/quora/2012/08/09/how-much-money-did-jonas-salk-potentially-forfeit-by-not-patenting-the-polio-vaccine/

[2] GSK is the merger of 17 independent drug companies: Glaxo, Borroughs, Wellcome, Smith, Kline, Beecham, and Beckham being the most recent acquisitions. https://chewychunks.files.wordpress.com/2010/09/pharmeceutical-company-acquisitions-map.png

[3] http://ebolastories.wordpress.com/2014/10/24/leaked-documents-reveal-behind-the-scenes-ebola-vaccine-issues/

[4] http://www.sciencemagazinedigital.org/sciencemagazine/20141031C?folio=534#pg22

[5] http://www.phrma.org/sites/default/files/pdf/2013innovationinthebiopharmaceuticalpipeline-analysisgroupfinal.pdf

[6] http://www.plosone.org/article/fetchObject.action?uri=info%3Adoi%2F10.1371%2Fjournal.pone.0048135&representation=PDF

[7] http://news.sciencemag.org/africa/2014/10/tough-choices-ahead-ebola-vaccine-trials

[8] Our compassion, or 'humanity' as it is often called.

4: Why won't they stop air traffic to the affected countries? We need to quarantine these people!

It is seductive to believe that this will work, but it won't. Let's break down the problem so you can see why the "build a wall" strategy will endanger more people everywhere, especially Americans.

Earlier in the epidemic both Liberia and Sierra Leone flirted with a quarantines and national lock downs. On August 19, 2014 President Sirleaf Johnson addressed the nation, "All entertainment centers are to be closed. Video centers will close at 6 pm. There will be a curfew from 9 pm to 6 am. West Point in Monrovia and Dolo Town in Margibi are under quarantine under further notice."[1]

West Point slum in Monrovia sits on a beach jutting out into the ocean. This tumble of tin shacks and its 75,000 residents were isolated when army and riot police barricaded all exits one night. They even sent in the coast guard to stop any refugees sneaking away in canoes.

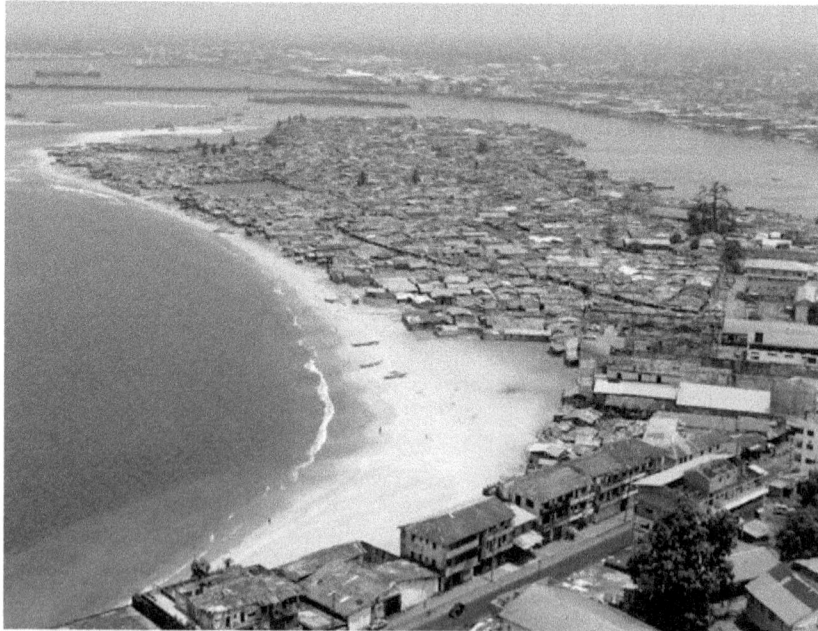

If their rationale was that isolating one neighborhood would contain the virus, it backfired. Here are local reports:

Steven became trapped inside West Point in a stroke of bad luck. He had been sleeping in his tailoring shop outside the slum for two weeks to avoid the crowded alleys amid the deadly outbreak. He returned to check on his family last Tuesday, and when he awoke Wednesday, the quarantine was in place. He couldn't leave. The military agreed to let him step outside the barricade for our interview and then he had to retreat. His face showed his anguish.

As we spoke, trucks exited West Point loaded with water. "Why is the water coming out?" I asked.

"They have raised the prices," Steven told me. "We cannot afford the water. Many can't buy the food."

Steven's life was disrupted by Ebola when his stepmother and father died from the disease. Three of his siblings are in a treatment center. He has no idea how they're doing.[2]

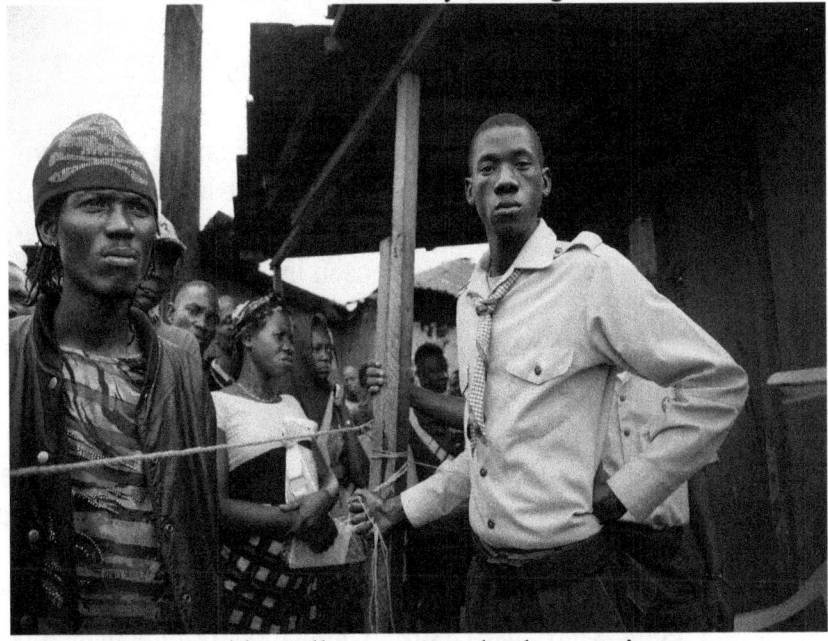

Pictured above: A thin, yellow rope marks the containment zone for the residents of West Point in Monrovia, Liberia. Nearby a boy scout stands guard.

Inside the barrier, there is desperation. Beyond, 20 people pleaded with me to share their story. We have nothing to eat, nothing to drink, no medical care, they said. They have been told they are under quarantine for 21 days to make sure they don't have Ebola. "Please let people know we are here," said a man concerned that his children have nothing to eat. "We only have tea."

"They hand out rice and beans," Steven says. "But how do we eat it without coal to burn to heat the water?"[3]

The WFP had been distributing food, but not enough for everyone. Everybody lost any trust they had for their government.

A few days later President Johnson Sirleaf visited.

"We suffering! No food, Ma, no eat. We beg you, Ma!" one man yelled at her as she visited West Point, surrounded by concentric circles of heavily armed guards, some linking arms and wearing surgical gloves.

"We want to go out!" yet another pleaded. "We want to be free, Mama, please."

Health experts warned her that quarantines work in villages and rural areas, but not in dense slums where tens of thousands of healthy people are trapped with sick ones, who can't get treatment. Instead President Sirleaf Johnson listened to her army, who advocated it.

Not only were citizens "crammed into crumbling shacks" like animals, the walls were porous. The checkpoints were futile:[4]

People are swimming in and out of the Ebola quarantine zone in this seaside capital. One man slips out every day to reach his job at a Western embassy. Another has turned his living room into a tollbooth, charging others to escape through his apartment at the edge of the cordoned area. Countless others have used a different method: bribing their way out with fees that soldiers determine according to a person's appearance, circumstances and even gender.

Within a week, the residents rioted in anger. Young men hurled rocks and stormed barbed-wire barricades. Soldiers responded with live rounds, driving them back. They overran a school that was being used as an Ebola holding center. Others dumped the highly contagious corpses of Ebola victims into the ocean to avoid handing them over to the government's body-collection teams.

In Dolo, the other town quarantined, people wore a paper tag on their collars bearing their body temperature, recorded twice a day. This community measure aimed to encourage trust in an area where people have died from Ebola and the fear of infection was palpable.[5] One resident said:

> We can see the trucks bringing the food but not everyone is getting it for now. Like us: we don't even have a ticket yet so we don't know when we will get the food. Until then, we have to rely on our family members out there to bring us food.

> They don't allow us to go anywhere. We are only allowed to go and stand at the (checkpoint) and family members from elsewhere can come there to bring us food and other things we need.[6]

Quarantines create distrust between citizens and the government. And this distrust creates more chaos, that leads to more harsh laws that make no sense and cannot be enforced. It is a vicious cycle illustrated by the anti-bicycling law passed in Makeni to deal with Ebola:

> September 29th, 2014: Rumors spread about the Ebola outbreak ending in Makeni, Sierra Leone.

> Youth on bikes rolled through town shouting, "Ebola don don, si tan to kuru yei pa Ernest o po mar su" which translated means "we thank God and president Koroma that our country is free of Ebola." Local authorities argue that since these rumors were spread by bike riders, they ought to ban bike riding, so they did. Three weeks later the minister lifted the biking ban and instead regulated bikes: bikes must be licensed, insured, and registered; no underage riders allowed; riders now need a license; and riders are only allowed to travel between 7am and 7pm.[7]

At an Ebola case management in Kenema, workers threaten to lay down their tools and strike following a four week delay in receiving their paychecks. They're still waiting.[8]

In Freetown, burial teams go on strike over lack of any prophylactic protective equipment (PPE) being provided to them, and not receiving pay for this hazardous work. And reports continue to come in of dead bodies not being picked up. Finally after a week of delays, the ministry paid up and they resumed work.

Sierra Leone's tried a three day national "lock down" to deal with Ebola. No one could go outside except medical personnel and police:

"My father, Pa Tengbeh, was without food for the past five days because we have been in quarantine and nobody is allowed to move from one place to another. We are poor. We get food from our farm work but the government has deployed police all over, but have not provided us with any food. This led to the death of my father."[9]

"I don't have any food because I am a disabled person and I don't have any way to get my food. We hope that we can get food through the government, who made a statement that disabled would have food. But where I am we don't have anything like that. I didn't eat anything today. I didn't get anything."

The quarantine didn't work. Ten days into it the government lifted it and tried something else. But the people of West Point learned their lesson. They started self-organizing and finding their own solutions:

MONROVIA, Liberia—Two months after Liberia's largest slum fought a government-imposed Ebola quarantine, residents are in a desperate push to conquer the deadly virus—with or without the government's help.

Ebola is still spreading through West Point, but so are changes to habits and traditional practices that offer a glimmer of hope. The behavior shift is also key to the international effort to contain the disease.

When the lockdown ended and international aid organizations poured into West Point with bleach, rubber boots and information, community leaders decided they needed to take action fast.

Prince Mambu, the head of a community group called Health Education, Sanitation and Sensitization Group, started going house to house talking with people who have had contact with victims. It is now routine. He reminds his neighbors to stay in their houses and asks about symptoms.

"I ask them, 'Do you have a headache?' But also I watch their eyes. Sometimes they say no but if I detect that they look weak, I will report it to the others. If they are willing, I will call for an ambulance," Mr. Mambu said.

22-year-old Mechie Seih told charcoal seller Mamie Kollie how to lower infection risk if a family member falls ill: "You put clean plastic bags on your hands. You wear a thick jacket with long trousers. You put shoes and socks on your feet."

Ms. Kollie nodded. She is being careful: Already outside her shop is a bucket of chlorinated water for washing hands. A woman selling dried fish nearby said she had stopped eating meat from animals like monkeys and rodents—commonly called bush meat—a suspected source of infection. A few doors down, a barber said special body-collection teams are now receiving calls from families when someone dies.

Pharmacist Doris Nyenkan says she now tells customers complaining of fever to get tested for Ebola. She also now stays a few feet away from customers and washes her hands at least once an hour.

"People clean their homes every day now. Now they are washing their hands, buying this gel," Ms. Nyenkan said, pointing to a bottle of hand sanitizer. "Before Ebola you didn't see people doing such things."

Tolbert Nyenswah, the head of the Liberian government's Ebola response, applauded West Point as one of a few Monrovia neighborhoods where residents have taken charge of the effort.

"They have their own active case finding, and they are quarantining households and checking for strangers. If people are sick, they report that to the call center," Mr. Nyenswah said.

People realize they would have been much worse off had they waited on the government to intervene.

"During the quarantine, medical teams were not coming here. There were no ambulances, things were just terrible here," Mr. Mambu said. It is better now, but the government is still too slow to respond: Ambulances sometimes take a day to arrive, he said.

Now, when West Point residents need an ambulance, many call Kenneth Martu —who works for a U.S.-funded charity called More Than Me. They used to run a school for West Point girls before the Ebola outbreak. Now, it pays for nurses to do rounds in West Point and provides lunch for Ebola response workers, in addition to sponsoring the ambulance service. Martu says they average about 10 ambulance calls a day.[10]

That's a dramatic turnaround and a testament to the power of local leaders to manage a crisis when the public comes to terms with reality. West Point is managing cases better than the national government could, while international donors provide supplies and training - but don't dictate who does what.

Meanwhile, many American bloggers like this one were spouting their views in favor of quarantines, but with no real understanding of the consequences[11]:

If we know the incubation period is 21 days, why not quarantine health workers returning from West Africa for 21 days to make sure they are free from the virus? That may be inconvenient for the volunteer, but as a healthcare worker they would understand what exposing the virus would mean to the general public. Simple precautions for a not so simple problem.

But that blogger answered his own question in the same post:

He was at a bowling alley on Wednesday and traveled via subway and taxi. It appears he just started showing symptoms Thursday morning, which according to what we know now is the only time the virus is contagious.

As soon as this returned Ebola worker started showing symptoms, he voluntarily admitted himself to isolation and quarantine. I suspect it is because he understood that hiding it would jeopardize the global response to Ebola. But he is exceptional. Few people beyond the front lines of this epidemic have ever thought about how their choices affect the strangers around them. They don't really accept that treating an epidemic in Liberia protects people in America, and they certainly don't understand the personal sacrifice that a blanket quarantine or travel ban would be asking each traveler to make.

Quarantined individuals cannot work. The average American worker uses 12 vacation days a year[12] and 25% of employees receive no vacation days at all, so imposing a mandatory 21-day quarantine on all travelers could cost a many their jobs.

If a man of Liberian descent returns home to America after visiting relatives in Liberia, only to face a 21-day quarantine, during which time he earns no wages, he is likely to avoid being honest about where he is coming from. He will take land transport to the nearest country outside the travel ban and fly from there. Or he will fly to Europe, switch airlines, and lie about visiting Liberia on his entrance forms. All of these are "simple precautions" he is taking to avoid the "simple precautions" imposed on his life. Any rational person would do the same if he or she had no symptoms of Ebola.

The people most in love with the idea of quarantines feel they're being pragmatic. Because they don't trust their government to check temperatures and regulate travelers properly, they think that unconditionally refusing all West African travelers entry would be easier and safer. Instead it would simply create a much larger West Point scenario. People would find another way in, but this time we wouldn't be able to trace their path. Strict barriers create incentives for people to avoid giving the system the information it needs to treat the problem. The repercussions are extensive and complex. It would endanger more people. We've already seen that those who don't trust their government become very dangerous when placed under quarantine.

It took Liberia only 10 days to realize the folly of a quarantine; I doubt America would reverse this bad policy until after Ebola started popping up in surprising places all over the country.

When faced with what real people are most likely to do under a threat of quarantine, the most effective approach is the pragmatic one we are already trying. These impractical proposals come from an attitude about this threat that vastly overestimate the effectiveness of laws, regulations, and police actions to control a population. It is a misjudgment common to both liberals and conservatives. For example, take apartheid in South Africa: Townships (African worker camps) were planned communities with walls around them and just two exits. This was intentional. The government wanted to isolate threats when (not if) a riot began. They expected life to be hard inside the walls, and they discounted the lives of the people inside. Would police stop looting and raping inside the walls during a riot? No. The effect of building townships in this way was to permanently increase crime and decrease prosperity for people living there, beyond what an open settlement of poor workers would have experienced. A walled-in community with two exits has less commerce and fewer jobs to offer. If we attempt to quarantine off whole countries, we will just amplify the township problem on a global scale, and we actually increase the unchecked spread of Ebola. Liberia's largest foreign employer, Firestone, is a role model because chose to do the opposite:

Firestone Tire [in Liberia][13] detected its first Ebola case on March 30, when an employee's wife arrived from northern Liberia. She'd been caring for a disease-stricken woman and was herself diagnosed with the disease. Since then, Firestone has done a remarkable job of keeping the virus at bay. It built its own treatment center and set up a comprehensive response that's managed to quickly stop transmission. Dr. Brendan Flannery, the head of the U.S. Centers for Disease Control and Prevention's team in Liberia, has hailed Firestone's efforts as resourceful, innovative and effective.

Ed Garcia, Firestone's general director, was quoted as saying, "None of us had any Ebola experience." They did have experience in acting decisively to manage tricky situations. They worked to clear out buildings and set up an isolation ward. They immediately quarantined the woman's family and prevented the spread of infection to anyone else at Firestone, including those who had cared for the infected woman. So a quarantine works in specific instances, on a small scale, and on a temporary basis. But any permanent and unconditional travel ban would make this epidemic spread faster.

[1] http://www.frontpageafricaonline.com/index.php/news/2717-ebola-curfew-liberia-announces-9-6-restrictions-west-point-quarantined
[2] http://abcnews.go.com/Health/inside-slum-cut-off-ebola-outbreak/story?id=25149920
[3] http://abcnews.go.com/Health/inside-slum-cut-off-ebola-outbreak/story?id=25149920
[4] http://ebolastories.wordpress.com/2014/08/
[5] http://wfp.tumblr.com/post/98306237478/life-under-ebola-quarantine-in-pictures-as
[6] http://news.yahoo.com/resentment-simmers-liberias-ebola-jail-town-111547180.html
[7] http://ebola.onourradar.org/2014/10/13/the-ban-of-bike-riders-okada-has-been-lifted-on-the-11th-of-october-in-the-city-of-makeni/
[8] http://ebola.onourradar.org/2014/10/13/workers-at-the-ebola-case-management-centre-at-the-government-hospital-in-kenema-have-threatened-to-down-their-tools-today-following-the-non-payment-of-their-allowances/
[9] http://ebola.onourradar.org/2014/09/27/the-late-pa-tengbeh-was-without-food-for-the-past-five-days-this-led-to-the-death-of-my-father/
[10] http://newstfionline.tumblr.com/post/100985142602/liberian-slum-takes-ebola-treatment-into-its-own-hands
[11] http://freevoter.com/2014/10/23/ebola-in-nyc/
[12] http://en.wikipedia.org/wiki/Annual_leave
[13] http://thefederalist.com/2014/10/20/ten-ways-the-public-sector-is-failing-and-the-private-sector-is-succeeding-against-ebola/

5: Why has it spread in Liberia and Sierra Leone but has been stopped in Guinea, Nigeria, and Senegal?

When Patrick Sawyer, a 40-year-old Liberian civil servant, realized he was sick and suspected Ebola, he flew to Nigeria in search of a good doctor he knew. Treatment options were limited in his home country, and being well-off and a bureaucrat to boot, he was used to flouting the rules. He probably bribed his way past the temperature checkers, was reportedly contagious on the plane, and collapsed in the airport on arrival. His condition rapidly deteriorated before he died, taking the life of his doctor with him. In the months that followed, 20 more people died before the outbreak was contained.

The outbreak in Nigeria was contained in spite of the huge numbers of people exposed to Patrick for two reasons: First, Ebola is difficult to catch. Each person typically infects two others, and not twenty others, because it requires human contact with tears, urine, semen, blood, vomit, and other fluids but notably not sweat. None of the people aboard Patrick's plane were at great risk beyond the person next to him. The other reason is that Patrick - a Liberian - traveled to meet one and one only person in secret - his doctor. This necessarily meant that he avoided contact with other people. Had he been traveling to a conference, funeral, or other family gathering the results would have been quite different.

The next West African country to confirm a case was Senegal, about a month later. In this case it was a university student who had been exposed and left the country while under surveillance. He traveled from Guinea to Dakar by land in search of better treatment, and did not disclose that he might have Ebola when he arrived. Having made that trip myself - more than 40 hours sitting with 39 of your closest pals in a passenger van that would normally hold 12 people in the United States, it is amazing that nobody else reported cases along his path.

Ebola cases appeared in Mali the following month. In this case the two vector patients were a two-year old girl whose father had worked for the Red Cross in Guinea and died of Ebola, and an

Imam (Muslim cleric). No other West African countries have reported cases.

What do the people that crossed the barriers of the epidemic in Guinea, Sierra Leone, and Liberia have in common? They are all people with status, privilege, and money. It takes money to travel - and so the people at greatest risk for spreading Ebola are those with the means to travel. More importantly, people who are used to flouting rules when it suits them are more likely to spread disease. Corruption and the spread of Ebola are correlated. Looking at a map of the region you might wonder why Ebola hasn't yet appeared in closer countries, such as Ghana. Ghana and Senegal are known to have the best governments and the lowest corruption in the region. Having a culture within civil servants that doesn't bend the rules and ask for bribes is a major deterrent to the spread of Ebola, it turns out.

This is the essence of a fragile state - that those with power (politicians, policemen, doctors, Imams, and rich people) get what they want. For this reason, another strategy to stopping Ebola is to change the bribery culture in neighboring countries. Hence, closed borders will actually remain closed. Liberia and Sierra Leone are fragile states in part because the central government is too corrupt to accomplish anything. Mali had a civil war in 2013 and is also a fragile state. Nigeria is a major trading hub and one of the most corrupt countries in the world. If this outbreak is not contained soon, it is likely that Nigeria will have a re-emergence of Ebola because its police are used to accepting bribes. But the lower levels of corruption in Senegal and Ghana will enable civil servants in those places to track travelers and stop infected people more effectively.

6: What would a global quarantine look like?

If Ebola infected on the order of 100 million people worldwide, global commerce would mostly stop. Daily activities would slow to a crawl. Schools would close at first, then switch to complete virtual learning with video conferencing after 6 months. Offices would go virtual too, with essential work being done from home or by minimum staff. People would avoid contact whenever possible with co-workers and customers and many types of delivery services would grow. You might imagine the government converting postal workers into a safe and heavily policed workforce with long hours, hazard pay, and constantly suited up. The Internet, electricity, water, and public works would continue to operate. Power plants would operate on lock-down, with three shifts of personnel living inside the plant for weeks, sleeping on cots in hallways, receiving food by delivery. Public servants (police, fire, medics) would protect themselves with gloves, surgical masks, safety glasses, and tyvek or hazmat suits, depending on the level of likely exposure to the disease. New temporary hospitals would appear in suburbs to meet the increased demand. Governments would declare a state of emergency and impose martial law. Travel restrictions would be localized then expand incrementally until just about everyone was isolated. If you can imagine a government that is a pure police state with a 24/7 curfew and house arrest for the masses, that's a good approximation of what the world would look like if Ebola infected millions with unabated growth. These predictions are simple extrapolations of what has already happened in West Africa.

This kind of doomsday scenario is useful for illustrating how seemingly small decisions become blunders and eventually snowball into genocidal policies. A harmless decision to bad travelers from West Africa - like Australia just did - could yield an unmanageable situation where Ebola is spread from unknown carriers. Because it cannot be contained, the next approach is a national lock down, like they tried in Sierra Leone. This puts a barrier between people and the basic supplies they need to survive.

It is nearly impossible to ensure that everybody gets what they need, and soon you have rioting, which calls for more police crackdowns, which further disrupts the system. It ends in one of two bad situations - either something that can hardly be called a society, or an insiders-outsiders divide with the rich and powerful protected and sustained behind walls and the rest left to fend for themselves. An epidemic without a healthcare system that attempts to treat everybody discriminates at best (if random) and is genocide in the worst case (if leaders choose which groups get abandoned without treatment, food, etc.)

The central thesis of this book is that Ebola is a crisis that brings out the best in good people, or the worst in other people. And a corollary to that is this: It is far easier to be a good person if you are willing to accept that the world's problems are complex. If you can accept the challenge of being more thoughtful, empathetic, and scientific, if you are willing to co-create the rules for how society treats its most vulnerable - the people in West Africa in this case - you'll be a hero. People who lead don't need titles. They just need to listen, think, empathize, and understand science. That last one leads me to the question most often asked by our least scientifically literate citizens in the next chapter.

7: Will Ebola become airborne?

No.

In October of 2014 I did a reddit ask-me-anything (AMA) live chat[1]. Of the 79 questions I answered, this was the most common question people kept coming back to over the course of the day. And since just saying "no" didn't seem to satisfy any of the reddit readers, I'll instead provide you various with arguments people have used to say "yes" and examine each one critically.

First, the CDC[2] and other reputable medical websites[3] have said that Ebola can be spread by inhalation. But most readers are confused by the jargon. To avoid adding to the confusion, the CDC took this material down from their site but put it back up again after an outcry from conspiracy theorists. This "Inhalation" does not mean the virus is airborne in the way the flu virus is airborne. If an infectious person sneezes in your face, they transmit saliva and phlegm directly onto your skin containing any virus. A sneeze creates an aerosol of body fluid and ejects it in all directions at over 100 miles an hour. An aerosol is a mist of tiny water droplets in air. Ebola victims can release large, virus-laden droplets - if, for example, their vomit splashes on the floor. These droplets may strike people in close range or land on a wall or some other surface, where they can stay infective for hours.

If these droplets end up in your mucus membranes, such as your eyes, mouth, and nose, then the virus can easily enter your body. And in the laboratory, army scientists did infect a group of monkeys with aerosolized Ebola virus in 1995[4]. All of the exposed monkeys died. This experiment was repeated in 2012 by another research group[5] who caution that this is not a normal or efficient mode of transmission. In fact, even when infected pigs transmitted Ebola to macaque monkeys in separate cages, the monkeys never transmitted it to each other[6]. So in one sense it is true that Ebola can pass from host to victim via the air, but only so long as the virus is inside microscopic water droplets. This is why health workers in West Africa wear protective clothing and breathe through an air filter. Standing inches from someone dying of Ebola as they sneeze, cough, vomit, and cry carries a risk of infection through aerosolized fluid transfer. Unprotected people tend to be safe standing just a few feet away from an Ebola patient[7], and Ebola doesn't cause very much sneezing and coughing anyway. And fear profiteers selling air filters to protect you from Ebola are wasting your money. The aerosol from a dying person needs to contact you almost immediately to take hold, not settling on some doorknob[8] and drying up.

This makes sense in the context of evolution. Viruses that have co-evolved with humans for millions of years are going to invoke the kinds of symptoms that best transmit copies of themselves to other hosts. People with the influenza virus (the flu) sneeze and cough because influenza's genetic code is optimized for airborne transfer. Ebola affects body fluids and has the unique trait of remaining active for days after the host has died; this is probably the optimal way it has evolved to infect others. Ebola and influenza are so genetically different that it would take thousands of mutations in a precise order for one to resemble the other. You and every member of your family are more likely to win the lottery on the same day than you are to see Ebola become truly airborne in your lifetime.

The most effective way to get Ebola is through breaks in your skin, or touching a victim's blood, feces, vomit, tears, breast milk, saliva, urine or tears. Sweat carries no trace of the virus, and is not considered a vector, so shaking hands is not a real threat - though people in West Africa stopped shaking hands as a precaution. And don't forget, carriers of the Ebola virus who have no fever are not at all contagious.

People and newspapers have been exploiting this public confusion about aerosol inhalation, making Ebola sound like an airborne disease. The New York Post claimed CDC materials said it was possible for casual contact with a doorknob to infect a person[9]. This is theoretically possible, if a dying person vomited or drooled all over the doorknob. Hence all precautions medics are taking, wearing scary hazmat suits and breathing through air filters. Whereas you are very likely to be exposed to the flu this year by touching a bathroom doorknob, no one is likely to get Ebola this way.

For months conspiracy bloggers have been claiming there is a cover up and that "Ebola virus had mutated and become airborne." This is preposterous. If they wanted a mutation story to scare the public, researchers working with the H5N1 virus produced this startling result. H5N1 normally requires contact with an infected bird, but exactly 5 mutations in the right spots was sufficient to make it an airborne virus, at least among ferrets[10]. No human has been exposed to this lab strain yet. And a single mutation in H5N1 is sufficient to make our anti-viral drugs useless. These are examples of a virus that poses a serious future threat because it has a high mutation rate and requires little genetic change to become a deadlier strain. It will likely happen in our lifetime.

[1] http://reddit.com/r/IAmA/comments/2i3cyg/we_work_for_local_and_international_aid_groups/
[2] http://www.cdc.gov/vhf/ebola/pdf/infections-spread-by-air-or-droplets.pdf
[3] http://www.uptodate.com/contents/epidemiology-pathogenesis-and-clinical-manifestations-of-ebola-and-marburg-virus-disease?source=search_result&search=ebola&selectedTitle=1~11
[4] http://www.ncbi.nlm.nih.gov/pmc/articles/PMC1997182/
[5] http://www.nature.com/srep/2012/121115/srep00811/full/srep00811.html
[6] http://www.virology.ws/2014/09/27/transmission-of-ebola-virus/
[7] http://www.nytimes.com/2014/10/24/us/fallacies-are-spreading-as-readily-as-the-virus-has.html
[8] http://www.huffingtonpost.com/2014/10/30/cdc-ebola_n_6078072.html
[9] http://www.huffingtonpost.com/2014/10/30/cdc-ebola_n_6078072.html
[10] http://www.sciencemag.org/content/336/6088/1534.abstract?sid=c406c7ab-0f9e-4ef9-b0db-97dc2cd729f3

8: What is having Ebola really like? And what it is like for doctors to treat patients?

Phillip Ireland was a Liberian doctor who worked at JFK Hospital in Monrovia, contracted Ebola and survived. He tells his story:[1]

It started during an office meeting. I had a terrible headache. It was so strong that I thought I saw lights, something like lightning. I immediately left the meeting and went to the clinic. I took my temperature and found out I had a fever and the first thing that struck me was that I had Ebola. Previously, I had been treating two of my colleagues who had died from Ebola. So when I got home, I told my family to leave the house and go to a relative's home so that they could get stay away from me.

My mother decided that she would stay with me and she made her own personal protective gear. I locked myself in a room, while my family was getting ready to leave the house. I remember my little seven-year-old daughter, Precious, came and opened the door of my room. She just wanted to know what happened to her dad, why he was being locked away, what was going on?

For me, that was the scariest moment of the whole Ebola experience. Here was my daughter opening a door and exposing herself to this life-threatening disease. I told her that daddy was sick. And I started screaming at the top of my lungs for someone to come and take her away straight away.

Because there were no spaces in any of the Ebola treatment units around the city, my treatment began at home. I was fed nutritional milk and lots of food high in antioxidants like nuts and Moringa[2] leaves. But one evening my symptoms got so bad that I began to go into shock and was dying. They got an ambulance to take me to the Ebola Treatment Unit (ETU) and by the time we arrived there I had passed out.

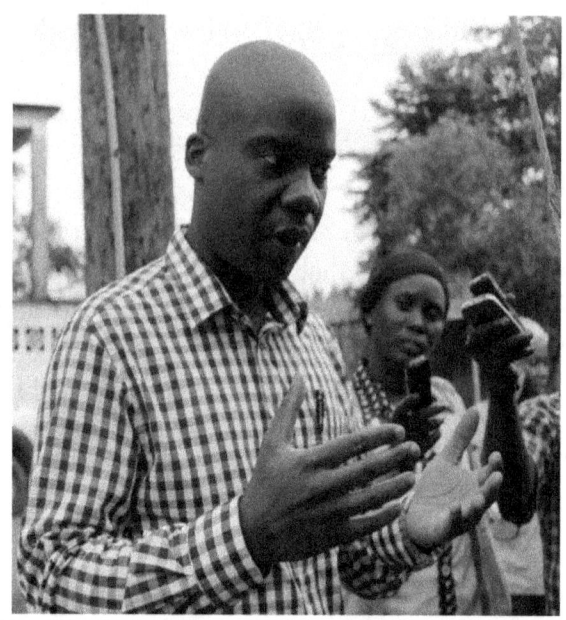

My whole experience in the ETU was like being face-to-face with death because there were dying people all around me. Even the best physicians we have in Liberia weren't enough. We had long periods of time where we would not see anyone - at first it was at 12-hour intervals. It was in those 12-hour windows that I saw a lot of people die.

Ebola is a terrible disease. It's a humiliating disease, it's debilitating. I remember that on the second night in the ETU, I had such bad diarrhoea and vomiting, that everyone thought that I was going to die in that period. I developed all kinds of complications. I had peripheral neuropathy - numbness, tingling and burning sensations in my feet and hands. I had pharyngitis. I had pneumonia. I had nausea. I had such terrible hiccups - at one point, I hiccupped with every single breath. It was so bad, I couldn't breathe.

While I was in the centre, I lost a colleague who was lying next to me in the isolation ward. He died during the 12 hour wait period and I spent the entire time lying there next to his dead body. I felt terrible. I tried to call for help and it took a while before someone responded to my call. They came in, checked that that he was dead, and then left. After another long wait, the body removal team came in and took away his body. It was a very sad and depressing experience. Another of my colleagues, another doctor, was also brought into the treatment centre while I was there, which made me feel very sad.

Through it all, I didn't bleed once which was a very good thing. I had been on the lookout for the bleeding because when you hear about Ebola, you automatically think about bleeding. The fact that I didn't bleed was comforting for me. After the third day in the treatment centre I started to feel a little better and walk around a little.

After I had been in the centre for 14 days, I was discharged. A lot of people turned up to see me walk out and welcome me. I always make a joke about this: as I came out, everyone who was there was crying, celebrating, and clapping - they all kept a safe distance though. As I got closer to them, they pulled further back from me. This continued when I went home.

People would come to see me, but they would stand very far away from me. Even my friends and close relatives. But I didn't have a problem with this - I didn't want to be the cause of anyone getting infected with Ebola.

I've been Ebola-free for two and a half months now. For probably a month after I came home, people were still afraid to come too close. Then my family started to come close - first my kids, my wife and my mother. Then other family members and friends began to follow suit. Although I know a few people who are still a little jittery around me.

A visiting doctor - James Appel - stationed at Adventist Hospital in Liberia kept a daily journal of his work treating Ebola patients, which he published online[3]. Here are some excepts:

The PA calls me to evaluate a patient who's come by taxi. We are sitting outside in the screening area to try and identify those with Ebola symptoms, so we can refer them to where they can be isolated and tested (the ELWA Hospital), without exposing our staff and patients.

An elderly woman sits motionless in the back seat, her face covered by a head scarf. Her legs are exposed revealing old sores on the ankle and foot with some edema. They say she hasn't pooped in five days. The belly is somewhat swollen but not tense. I remove the head scarf and she looks like death warmed over. My radar is on high alert. I can't take the risk. I tell the family there's nothing we can do. They try to protest and show me a torn slip of paper with some doctor's name and phone number on it with a note in chicken scratch saying "not suspicious for Ebola." That makes me more suspicious and I insist they leave. It's hard to do, my whole medical training screams "no!" but I know I have to protect the staff and patients and keep the hospital open so we can help those who can be helped. If we admit an Ebola patient, none of the staff or patients will come and many others will die who could be helped.

I go eat a quick lunch while they are decontaminating the room. I come back just in time to see the PA putting in a ten year old boy who is wearing only a ragged pair of shorts that are soaked in urine or other bodily fluids. I quickly learn that he was brought in urgently by his mom who carried him on his back and he's been vomiting with fever.

"GET HIM OUT OF HERE!" I yell. "THESE ARE EXACTLY THE CASES THAT WE ARE SCREENING FOR!"

Just then the mother let's out a wail. The child is dead. She grabs the boy and runs out. I continue to explain in a loud voice to all the staff that these are exactly the cases that are supposed to be screened and sent away. The PA's reply is that he was too sick to screen outside so he brought him in on a bed.

"He died immediately anyway so we didn't help him," I said. "We only put ourselves at risk."

A week later:

Maybe I'm starting to imagine things in my paranoia, but I'm beginning to think I can recognize an Ebola patient on sight. Maybe it's my intuition. Maybe I'm imagining it. I can start to see it in their eyes. They just have that look. The eyes kind of bulge out. They have a sort of blank stare. The inside of the eyelids are more red than normal. The surface of the eyes, the white part, the scleral conjunctiva seems to be a little edematous and not quite the right color: not quite yellow as in jaundice, but not quite white either. It's subtle.

Today when I go out to see this ten year old girl, in my mind I've already decided she has malaria. I go through the motions of asking all the screening questions and she sounds like she has malaria: headache, fever, loss of appetite, no vomiting or diarrhea. Instinctively, I check her eyelids to see if she has anemia like everyone else. Most of the kids have had very pale palpebral conjunctiva, but this girl's are bright red. It sets of warning bells in my head, but I ignore my instinct. It's probably malaria I tell myself. I don't want to send her to certain death of malaria by refusing her, so I let her come in against my gut feeling.

I hope the mistake doesn't turn out to be too costly.

We bring her into the ER and the nurses find an IV. As the nurse is taping the catheter in place she asks me if I've noticed the rash. She has a raised rash all over her arms and trunk and face. It doesn't look like anything I've seen before. I just gave her an Artemether shot in her muscle. There was no bleeding. Now I look back and some blood is pooling over the injection site. Jeff from the lab is right there. I ask him to go get a rapid malaria test and do it here at bedside. Meanwhile, we start the Quinine drip for malaria.

I look again at her conjunctiva again. They really are more red then normal. I'm starting to get a suspicious feeling. Sure enough the malaria smear is normal. And where Jeff pricked her finger is also bleeding more than normal. And she has a high fever. There's a reason they call it Ebola Hemorrhagic fever. Of all the suspicious cases we've had here, this is the first I've seen with bleeding. Of all the cases I've seen, this has to be the most suspicious for Ebola I've seen yet.

I call in the mother. She's dressed in some kind of police or security uniform. I explain that I'm suspicious of Ebola and they should take her immediately to either of the Ebola Centers: JFK government hospital or EWLA Hospital where Doctors Without Borders has set up shop. They leave immediately. We wash down everything and throw away anything that we may have touched. I run home, take a shower and wash my scrubs and put on new clothes. This is my closest brush with Ebola yet.

A few hours later, the mother is back with the girl in the back of the car.

"Dey look at de IV and say to take her back to where she bein' treated…"

Are you kidding me!? It turns out that neither place would take her. Both are overrun. Dr. Martin comes out and tries to call some colleagues who work at the Ebola treatment centers. No one is picking up. There just aren't enough isolation beds or tents or personnel or supplies or anything. They are turning away patients left and right. But to not even test? And to use the excuse that she is being treated elsewhere and turn her away because we left the IV in to help them out so they could treat her without the risks of starting another IV?

I do what I should've done before: I write out a referral explaining why we think she has Ebola. I tell them to go back and persist and don't let themselves be turned away. Dr. Martin also suggests a third hospital, Redemption which is supposed to be opening or already open as an Ebola treatment center. We don't know.

Obviously, the family is frustrated and turns away sorrowfully. Did she die? We'll never know. If there were only the resources to isolate all the suspicious cases and test them -- Then if they are negative, get them referred to a hospital such as our own which is treating non-Ebola cases and get them the malaria or other treatment they need. And if they have Ebola, there should be personnel, protective gear and IV fluids to treat them, not to mention the availability of experimental drugs known to help certain Ebola patients.

Instead, chaos, fear, suspicion, lies and death abounds in Liberia.

[1] http://www.actionaid.org.uk/about-us/voices-blog/2014/11/05/what-is-it-like-to-have-ebola-and-survive
[2] This leaf has proven medicinal and nutritional value and works as an antioxidant, among other things. It can even be pressed into cakes and used as a water filter. http://www.webmd.com/vitamins-supplements/ingredientmono-1242-moringa.aspx?activeingredientid=1242&activeingredientname=moringa
[3] http://ebolastories.wordpress.com/2014/09/19/ebola-liberian-doctor-journal/

9: What is life like under Ebola in West Africa?

This is the question that drove me to search for answers, and led to me writing this book. Everywhere I looked, I found almost no first hand accounts. The few sources I did find were the same people being re-quoted. Everything had been digested and sanitized by the Associated Press and Reuters. I wanted the raw reports, transcripts, and dialogues, but our news was missing local people telling their story in their own voice. I started calling people I knew in the region. They led me to other people working on the ground, which led to these reports.

From eboladeeply.org[1]:

Dorcas is 17 years old. Her mom contracted Ebola when treating a patient in the clinic where she was a nurse. Dorcas took care of her mom when she was sick at home. Her dad, her elder sister and her mom were all infected and admitted. At the hospital, after her mom and elder sister died, Dorcas was helping to take care of her dad - even in the ward where they were both sick. Her father eventually died. Dorcas survived. She is left with her two younger siblings, who have become her primary responsibility. She is now the breadwinner and without support might be forced to engage in risky behaviors to fend for herself and her family. She is also unsure of returning to school, as there is no one to take care of her or pay her [tuition] fees.

Unfortunately, her story is not unique. Many of the 30-plus girl survivors of Ebola told me varying versions of a similar story. Girls in Sierra Leone are typically the primary caregivers for sick relatives.

Creating a support system for these girls will be crucial. Creating Ebola survivors' clubs could be one way to help, a place for them to share their stories and get support. They could also be powerful role models for other girls.

Chernor Bah of eboladeeply.org goes on:

We have received reports of police officers - assigned to enforce the quarantine of households - sexually molesting young girls. Bear in mind that typically during school holidays, when girls are at home, there is normally a spike in sexual abuse and exploitation. Now you have communities that are shut down, with men and young girls home all day. No one knows when this is all going to end. As one girl put it to me, "It's not a very safe time to be a girl."

Amid the shock of the epidemic, the government and the donors basically instructed that all programs that were not directly dealing with Ebola be shut down, and that funds all be redirected to fighting the epidemic. So these nonprofits have for the most part been on the sidelines, watching.

Chernor Bah's last comment is not entirely accurate. At GlobalGiving where I work, we worked with 22 Liberian organizations that were running local projects that had nothing to do with health in 2014. Since August, all of them have redirected their efforts to fighting the spread of Ebola. Many foreign ex-pat workers left but the local staff at these organizations continued to work. These people are not "on the sidelines" at all, but retraining and refocusing on the emerging needs of each community during this crisis. The organization More Than Me[2] exemplifies the rapid pivoting that all organizations are doing now:

When President Sirleaf recommended on July 30th[3] that schools close, we had to follow suit for the safety of our girls, staff, and community. On that day, we gave care packages to the girls that included workbook pages to keep them busy and learning, medicine for fever and bacterial illnesses, Ebola awareness posters, health care referral forms, oral rehydration solutions, chlorine, soap, and rice. All students and staff also attended an awareness class led by doctors and staff from UNICEF, the IRC, and Ministry of Health. While the school is closed, all expat staff members are being relocated to the US.

We have been monitoring the situation on the ground through ongoing contact with other NGOs, government ministries, and our local staff. On August 22nd, our founder Katie Meyler flew from the US to Liberia to help fight Ebola in the West Point community, where the majority of our girls live. The following are excerpts Katie's blog - http://racingheartblog.tumblr.com/ - started when she arrived. Life in West Point slum, Monrovia, Liberia:

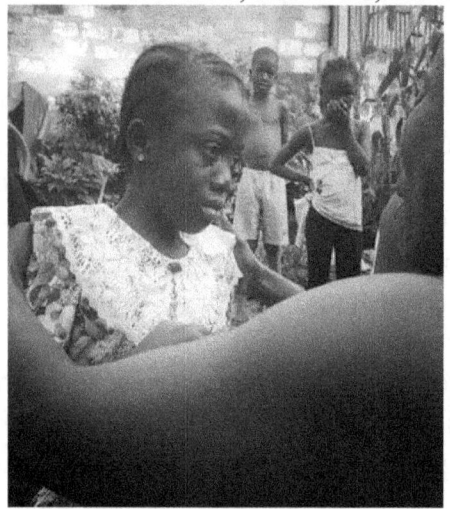

Josephine's 28 year old mom died. I was there when they told her. No one is sure what killed her yet. Ebola? Poison? Hard to say without testing. Josephine had been living at the @MoreThanMeOrg staff house with her aunt Esther because her parents were too poor to care for her. Jo kept asking to visit her mom but because of Ebola Esther didn't think Josephine should travel. Now she won't be able to see her mother ever again.

Josephine's family was forced to move. They have 30 days to find a new home. Without a paycheck they are worried and begging for us to hire them. Stories like hers are normal here.

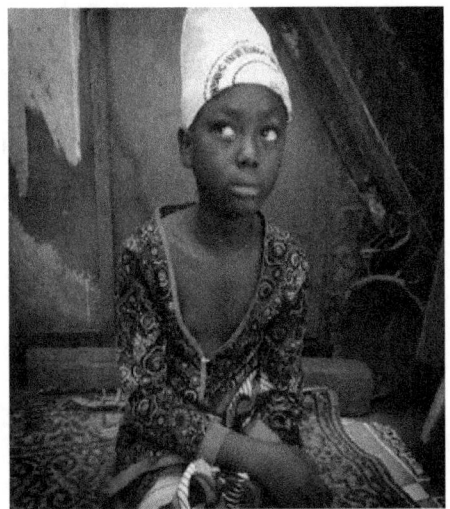

For hours, Sarah sat waiting for the ambulance. I got a call that this 10 year old child was sick. She has already lost her dad and her little 7 year old sister in October. Pray for Sarah that she will make it. We were able to give her a phone so her family could call to encourage her, and so that we can check up on her in the hospital. Sarah's sweet grandma was asked to leave because she couldn't hold herself together. Luckily, Sarah's mom was strong and in control in the midst of fear and chaos.

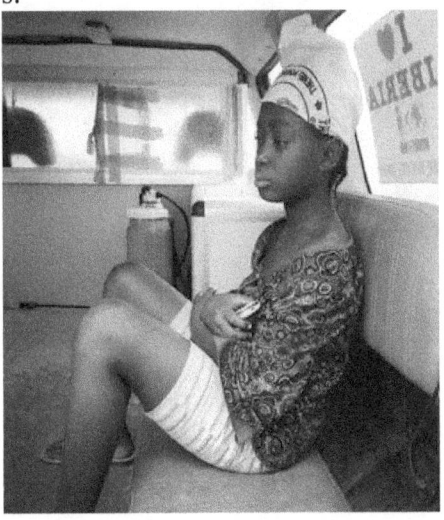

The Ambulance arrived, and the medic yelled to the onlooking crowd to get Sarah some drinking water. Sarah sat alone in the ambulance. This sickness isolates people. That's one of the worst things about it. None of her family could go with her to comfort her.

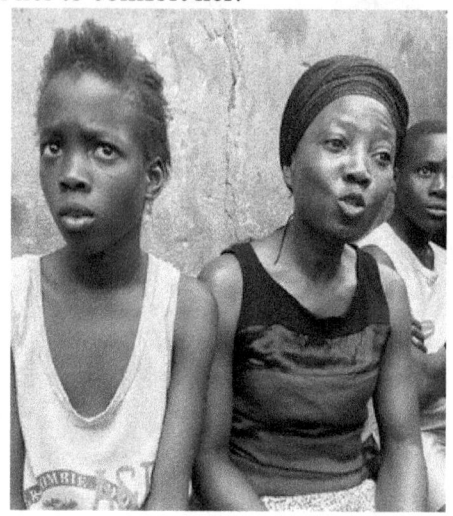

This little girl and her brother and sister lost their parents. The auntie is asking me to help her by taking the kids. I asked her, "If someone helped you support and empower her, would you could feel happy raising your sister's children?"

"Of course!" She said. This is reason #900 why More Than Me needs a boarding school.

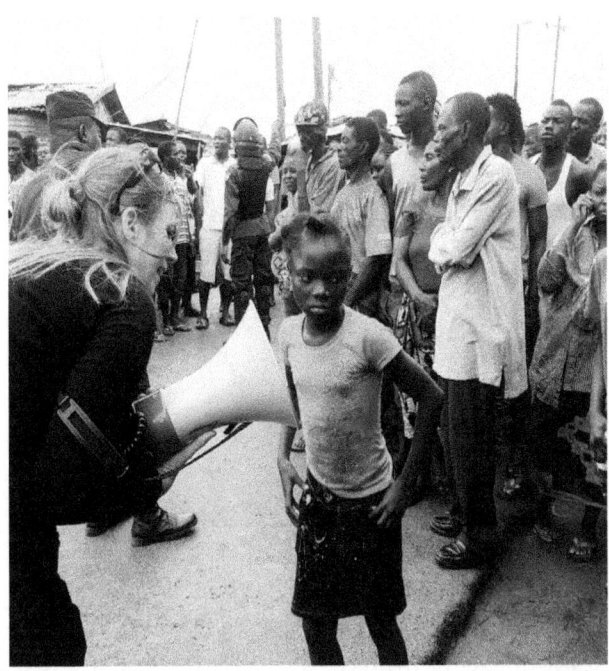

Rebecca tells me she has symptoms and is scared. I took my gloves off and let my hair down because I was leaving for the day. I wasn't scared, because she looked strong. We are bringing her meds and will keep a close eye on her. Obviously this is agonizing but we are doing all we can. Please pray for Rebecca with me.

The next day, I talked to local medical staff about serving West Point. Everyone I met was really lovely. There were 20 or 30 body bags with deceased people inside. I was scared but also at peace. This place has things under control.

Community leaders made the rounds in West Point and found 45 sick people in the areas they were able to check. Unfortunately, all of the clinics are at capacity and not able to receive people.

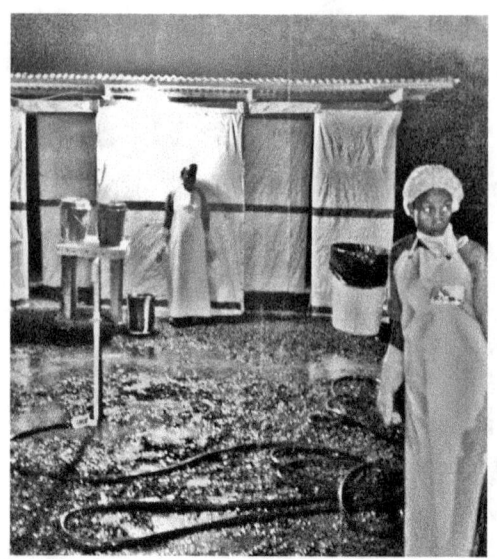

This is the bathroom in the Ebola treatment centre. You can see the floor is covered with feces and vomit. I heard a lady yelling for her baby from the sick ward. Her baby was tested negative and she was positive. The staff said she's a character and that those people tend to be more likely to live.

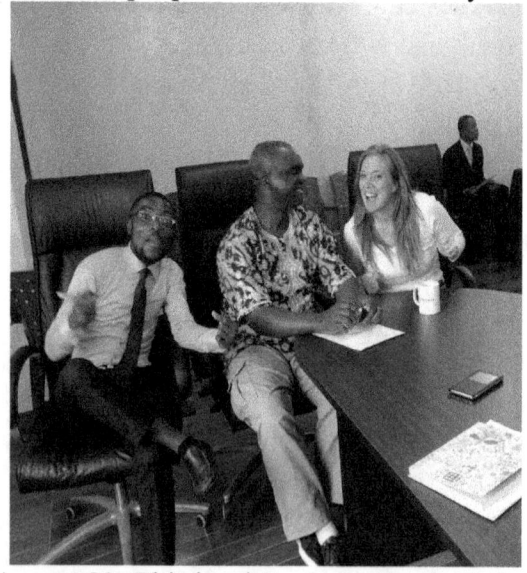

August 29: This is what emergency logistics planning looks like. Today I met with the honorable Tolbert, Assistant

Minister of Health. I asked if the Task Force Against Ebola could get their approval. This is a plan devised by local West Point leaders and NGOs for how to deal with the epidemic right now. We can't wait for the international community to swoop in and deliver a fix. He was friendly and supportive! Here's a picture of my notes:

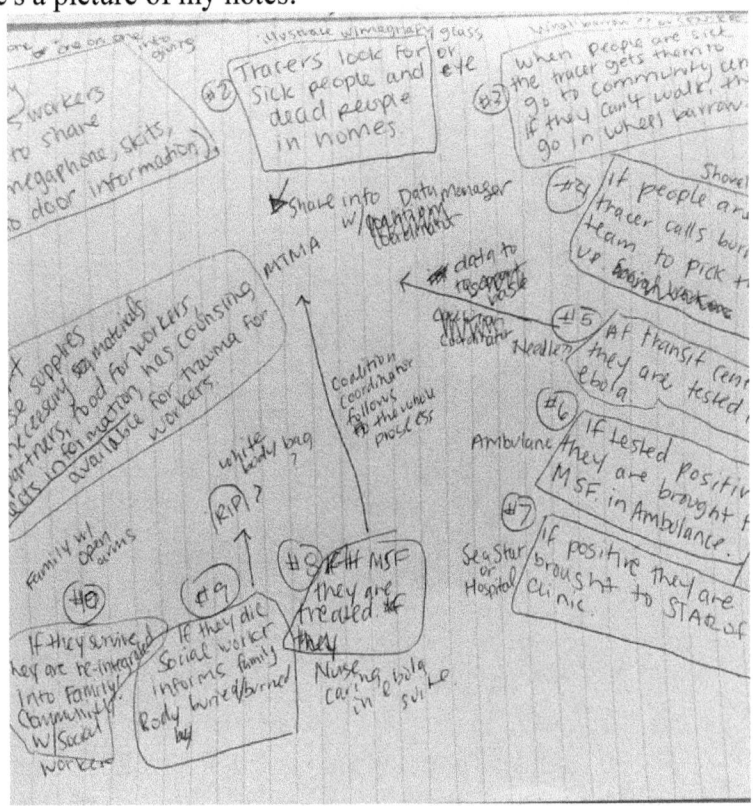

This sketch is now on More Than Me's website as a plan for a community response to the Ebola threat:

COMMUNITY BASED EBOLA-FREE COALITION

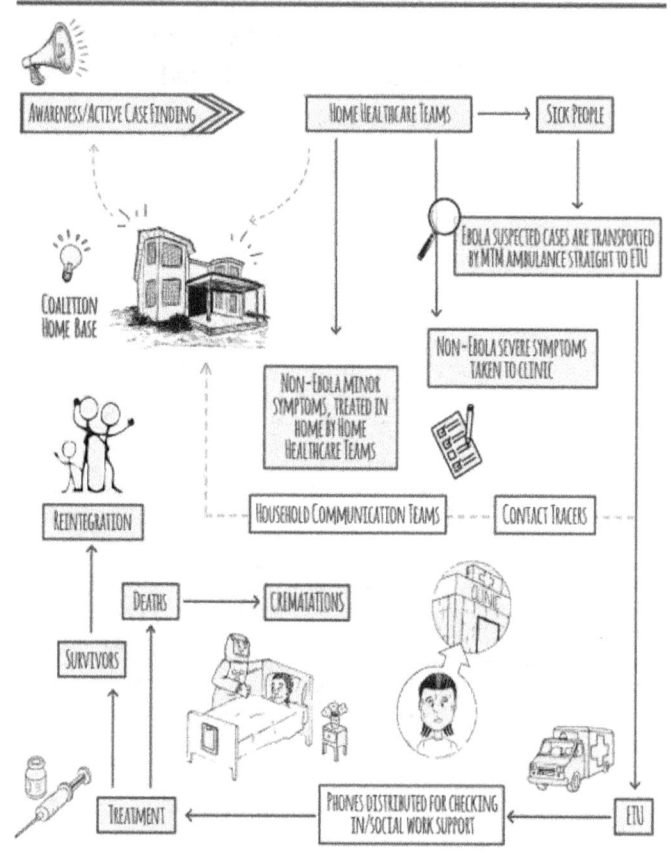

30 August: They stopped our car and took my temperature on the way to Cellcom to get a phone for our ambulance and burial team.

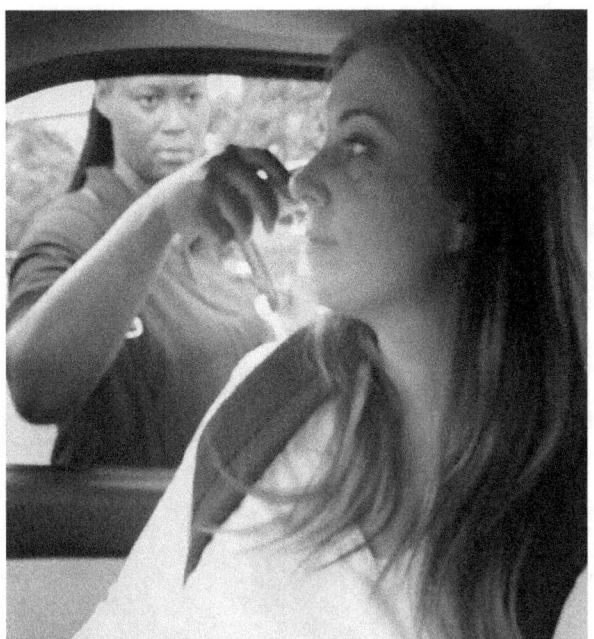

Everyone here thinks these temperature gun things are Ebola testers. They do seem like they could be, super sophisticated looking. We have one too. I asked her if I could take her temp back :)

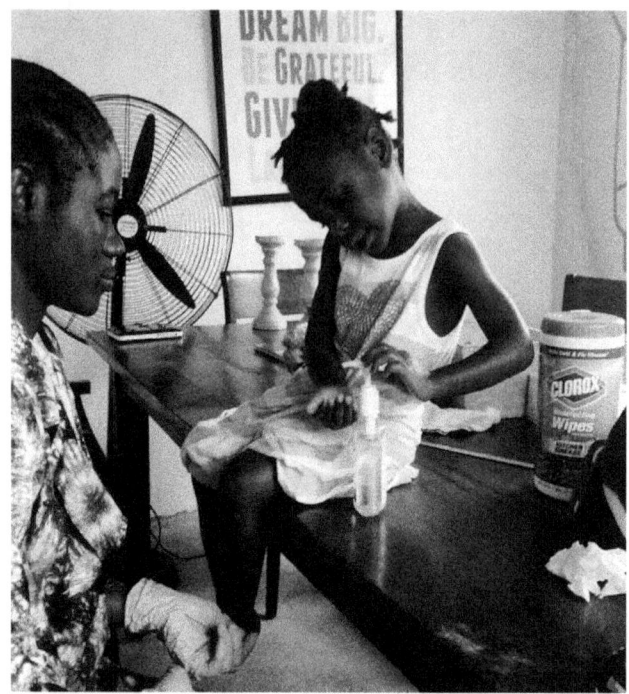

Little Pearlina is obsessed with washing her hands. She is not showing any symptoms. Today was day four. Yay!

8 September: This is my heart breaking, really. Just learned about the first person I knew first-hand to get Ebola. Dr. Sacra, an American doctor, fixed my leg after a motorcycle accident here back in 2006. He is the most humble, compassionate person. He was flown to Nebraska.

Today my neighbor lost her husband. I remember bringing them chlorine and fresh water. We sang and prayed together and provided them with Ebola facts. Today she still didn't know or understand how to get Ebola, or what her husband actually died of. My other neighbor's husband is in the Ebola treatment unit too. We discussed how she can help herself and family while they wait to hear from him. I hate Ebola.

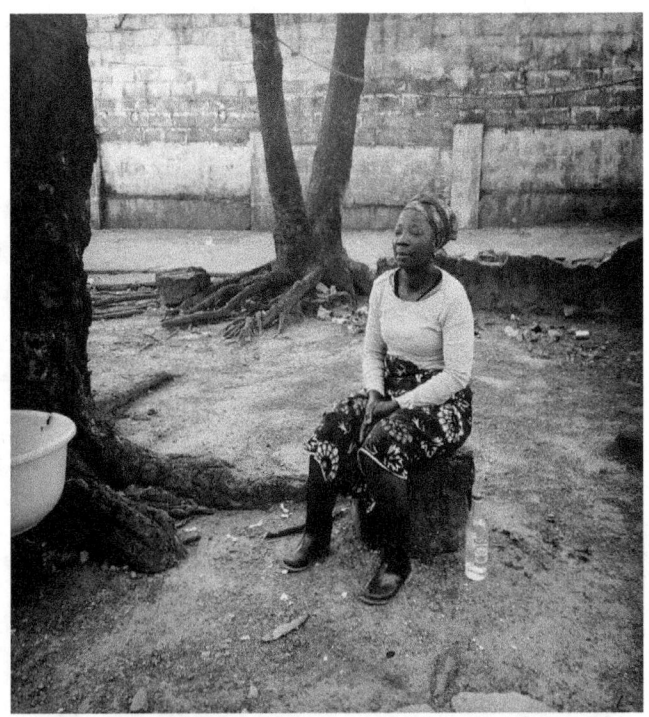

12 September: She is under quarantine in West Point. We talked a little. She said she's just sitting home for 21 days. She said, "you really did well for us, Katie." She was expressing how it's like the world and the government just abandoned her, leaving her and her family to die. She said the rice and food we were able to provide was helpful. Honestly, more than anything, I just want her to know she's not alone. That people do care, our team cares, I care. She's my neighbor.

The awareness teams meet at a church everyday where we being lunch and share challenges so we can solve them. At the meeting they adopted seven colors for seven different zones in West Point. I love it! Let's do it!

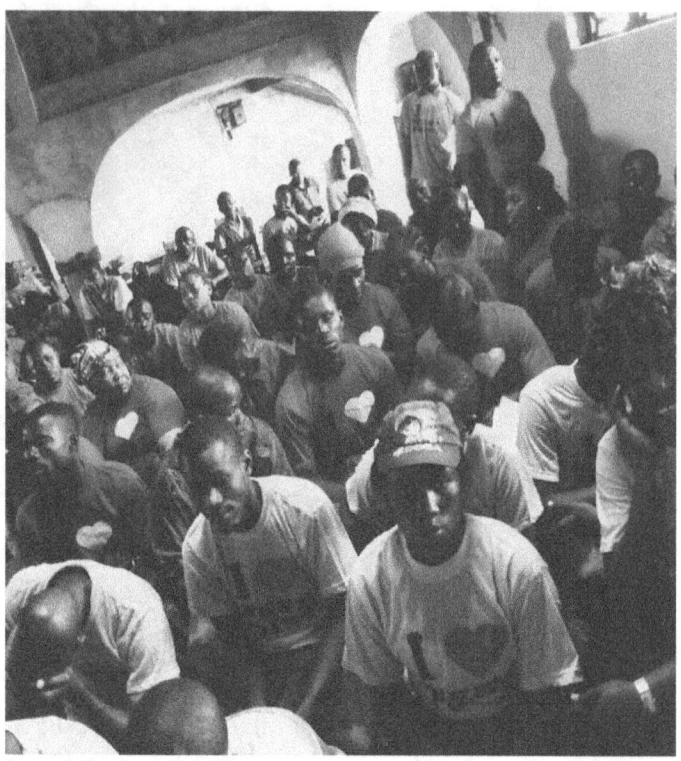

I heard from a credible source at a meeting that because things are so out of control here, we need a way to learn whether our messages are getting out to the community. I think I'll just tell people these three main points for now:
(1)   Don't touch fluids or sick people.
(2)   Wash hands with soap and water every 15 minutes
(3)   If you have sick people, isolate them, give them water, food, and use plastic to protect yourself.

We're thinking about offering incentives for the group with the best awareness of the message. I'll show up to different West Point zones and ask five random people what the ILoveWestPoint team just told them. The zone with the clearest knowledge gets an award - extra phone credit! We think it will encourage people to share the information better.

I met Gideon, a nurse at Redemption hospital. He explained his idea for an admitting system at the hospital.

There is currently none. He wants hospital bracelets. He explains that people are dying and there is no way to identify them to inform their families.

22 September: Kenneth our ambulance manager jumps out of the car and into the center of this fight to break it up. The food distributions in West Point are compassionate but somehow cause a lot of fighting and traffic jams.

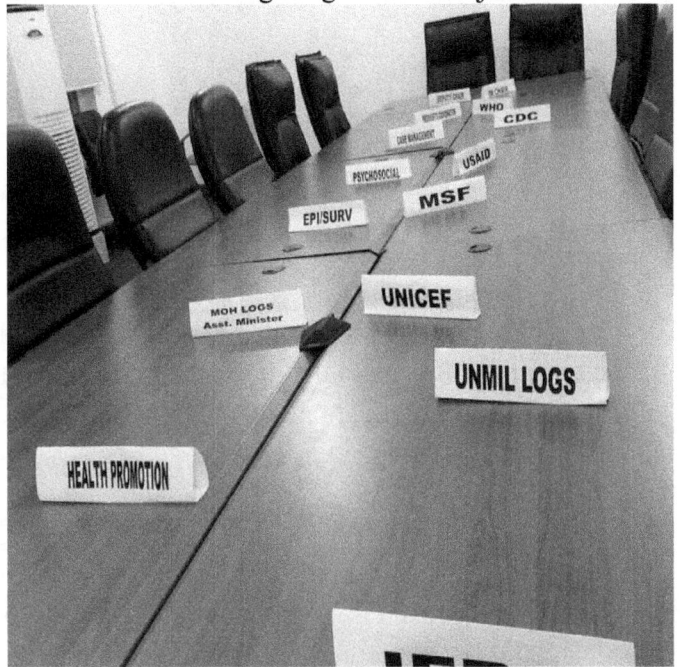

22 September: The voices at the table: MSF, UNICEF, UNMIL LOGS, HEALTH PROMOTION, MOH LOGS Assistant Minister, EPI/SURV, Psychosocial, USAID, CDC, WHO, UNCHR, Case management, Deputy Chair, Vice Chair. [Author's interjection: Where are the seats at the table for the people who appear to be doing the day-to-day work in West Point Slum?]

2 October: Teams of case finders are starting to pop up outside the city. I met with a group that organized themselves and started referring sick people to the authorities systematically. They were standing outside a school block

waiting to get paid. They had been working for free for three months.

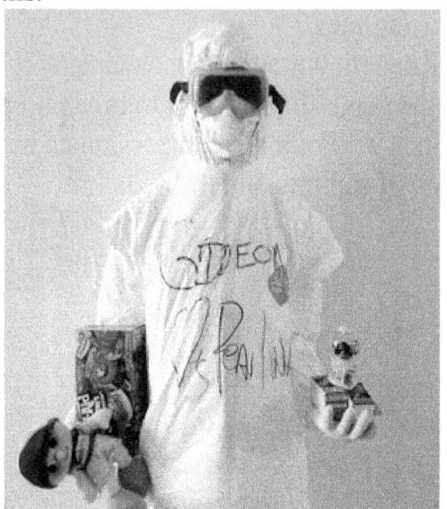

You all keep asking me about Pearlina. We fought hours of traffic and hot sun to get to the Ebola treatment unit on the edge of the city. We brought along crap loads of juice, vitamins, and toys for the kids. I wasn't getting any info when I called.

Even in person they aren't telling us anything. So, Gideon - the nurse who found her in the ambulance - suited up in full gear and wrote "Gideon loves Pearlina" on her vest, so Pearlina might recognize her. She is going into the Ebola Treatment Unit now to try to find Pearlina among the over 65 children in there. There she goes. Pray and wish and hope with everything you have she's fine.

3 October: We had 62 suspected cases in West Point two weeks ago and we have 0 cases as of today. The key to this was (1) nurses being able to differentiate between an Ebola suspect and someone having gout, and (2) having an ambulance to remove a probable Ebola case immediately.

6 October: We turned part of our school Library into a warehouse for medical supplies. Other ambulance teams keep showing up and asking us for basic gear to protect themselves.

These supplies save lives, but there is never enough. The next day I spoke with WHO about the issues at the Ebola treatment units. He said one of the clinics ran out of bleach.

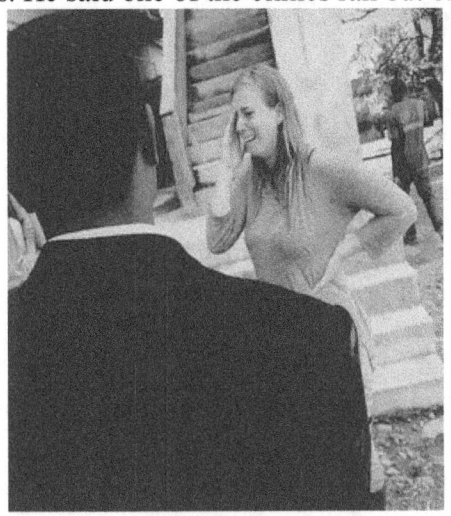

That same day I found out Esther had to leave. We are not an orphanage so she couldn't stay. That was really hard for all of us. She has a place at MTM Academy. I'm going to visit her today.

10 October: I went to check on Dede and her family at Island Clinic, an Ebola Treatment Unit, and see if they needed anything from our stocks. The workers were there demonstrating. Someone said they were replacing Doctor Atai, the woman running the place, and the workers said "If she goes, we all quit!"

I'm not sure why she was asked to go. I'll ask her tomorrow. Meanwhile around the corner a group of people who just beat Ebola were released onto the corner. They were just standing around the church beside Island Clinic. They had no ride home. I wanted to drive them home but my taxi said, no. It made me sad, but as messed up as it might sound, I'm happy they are alive to have that problem. Even problems are a privilege in some strange way in Ebola time.

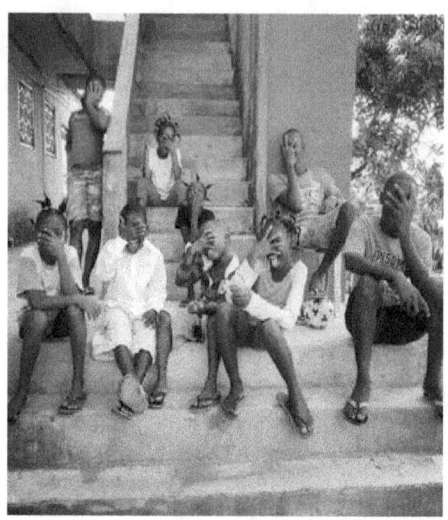

Nov 5, 2014: To protect their own identity, these children are covering their faces. All of them made it 21 days Ebola free but not all of them have a place to live now that their quarantine is over. The ministry of health is looking for a to place for them.

These days there are more children working than ever, because school has been closed for most of the year.

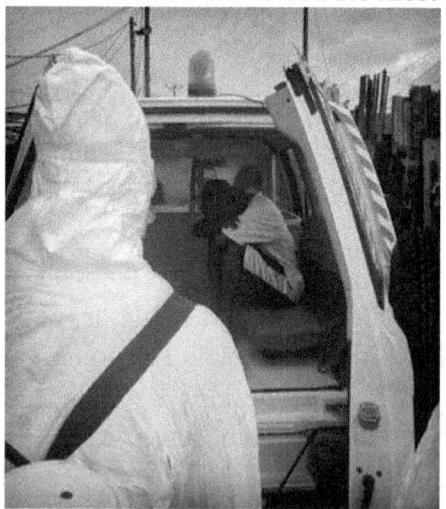

19 November 2014: I was in a town hall meeting with the elders, the women group, youth representatives, religious

leaders, and the clinic. This boy stands up, looks at me and says,

"I would not be alive today if More Than Me ambulance didn't come on time for me." Everyone clapped and started cheering. I think it hit me for the first time for real. We are literally saving lives. Our team is brave and I'm honored to be serving the Liberian people at their side.

From Kai Hopkins of Keystone Accountability[4]:

Outside the hospital gate crowds gather waiting for news, some cry, some pray, some shout to try and talk to loved ones inside. Round the corner at the morgue, it's a similar scene with crowds gathered, many in tears. Elsewhere life goes on. People sell their wares and walk on by, ignoring the commotion.

In Freetown the signs of the crisis are rather subtle. There are plenty of posters proclaiming that "Ebola is real", there are buckets of chlorine outside supermarkets and offices, and people take your temperature as you come and go - a reassuringly consistent 36.6°C. There is growing concern about a 'second crisis' as major public health issues like malaria are sidelined and the suspension of free maternal and child health care leaves many vulnerable. Fear or stigmatization prevents people from reporting possible new cases. One NGO manager said, "We are all interested in the apparent drop in reported cases in Liberia. Where once there were no beds, now centres sit empty. Why?"

Could stigma be affecting what we see?

Another aspect of the second crisis is the fear of an impending food shortage. Quarantines of Ebola houses, as well as broader restrictions on movement have hit all economic activity, especially around food, with the UN[5] warning that "in some areas, hunger has become an even greater concern than the virus". This invisible and deadly virus is leaving some very visible scars in a wide variety of places.

The future economic impact of Ebola is so large that the World Bank has already sent hundreds of millions of dollars to the region. There is no solution to an economy that grinds to a halt like this. The best we can hope to do is keep people alive and fed until they can start their lives over. Sadly, all of Africa is at risk. Ghanaians say, "what America sneezes, Africa catches a cold." What it means is that attitudes of ordinary Americans have a real effect on the continent. Many African businesses thousands of miles from Ebola are going to close this year. Here is an example from one blog:

Hi Mukwano ,

Hope the family is doing well. Ebola is killing our business. Greetings from my family. Wish you all the best. Big hug goes to all my friends. Kind regards, Ezra.

From Kampala, Uganda (over 3000 miles away from nearest Ebola)[6]

The blogger continues:

I have been friends with Ezra now for over a decade and have watched him grow his tour company from a single vehicle with a few clients a year to a thriving business offering safaris and vehicle rentals to hundreds. Ebola, a disease that is farther from Kampala than it is from Paris, is costing the tourism industry throughout African billions of dollars and crushing small tour operators like Ezra.

Another way to see how our attitudes shape what the world sees on an issue is through algorithms that summarize Internet trends. I wrote a program that scrapes the Internet and archives everything Ebola related. I used it to produce wordtree maps like this one:

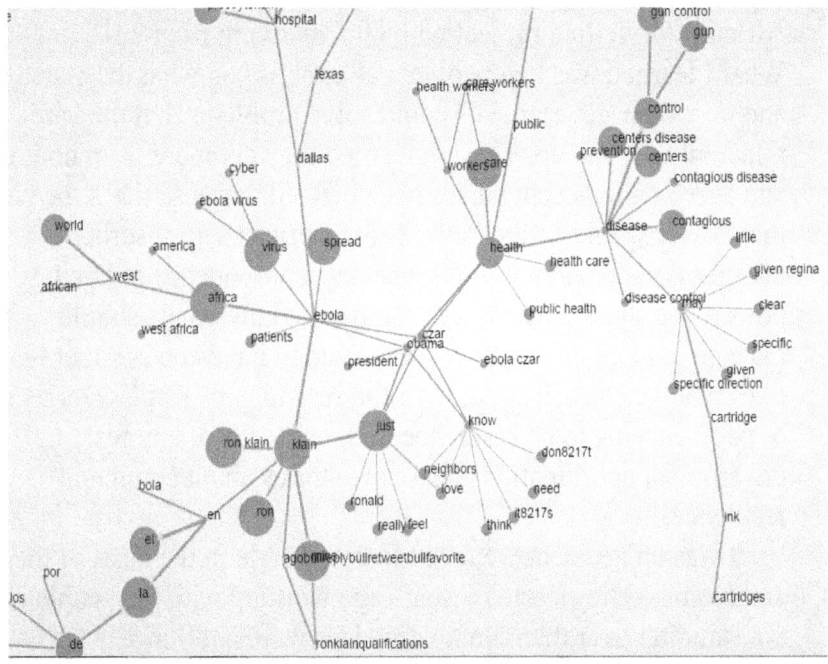

What this map reveals is that the Internet was almost entirely Americans talking about their fears of Ebola, not chatter from people directly affected. The map (from all wordpress content posted on October 18th, 2014) shows that petty American issues like the newly appointed Ebola Czar, ink cartridges, and gun control were drowning out any local voices[7]. Since only blog posts tagged by their authors with the keyword #Ebola were included, these wandering themes are much more common than anything else. Distractions are the "signal," not the "noise." The ease with which these maps get overwhelmed by blogs about American fears gives me reason to say that Americans are quantitatively the most self-absorbed, loud-mouthed, skittish people on the planet. If we were better listeners, at least a fraction of posts would contain narratives from people like those that Katie Meyler has been helping in Liberia.

For the last few year's it's been my work to figure out how to bring as much of this first-hand narrative from the poorer citizens of the world to the attention of those in power. I ran an East

African storytelling project with GlobalGiving from 2010 to 2013. What I learned was that people are "experts" on what they need and how their governments could solve problems, but they are reluctant to speak up. They've learned they get more from nodding and agreeing to accept what's been offered, because that's the way that Power speaks to the Poor. The American self-absorbed blogger isn't an anomaly - it's a natural consequence of having power. We share how we feel and debate how others should manage our country because we're used to have control over our lives that we can affect our own future. Many of Katie's stories are of people trying to be resilience in the absence of any real government coordination. These are stories about community resilience.

It was no accident we find More Than Me in the heart of the community. They started 9 years ago working with the people and not standing over them. In the timeless words of Sun Tzu:[8]

"Come among the people.
Live among them.
Work with that they have.
Build on what they know.
And when the work is finished, they will say,
'we have done this ourselves!'"

There has never been a better credo for fighting poverty, nor a better description of resilience. There are many technical ways to stop Ebola, but underneath every successful strategy is an appetite to empower resilient communities in precisely the way that Katie has. She knows very little about Ebola, but a whole lot about people.

[1] http://www.eboladeeply.org/articles/2014/11/6494/ebola-women-chernor-bah-impact-girls-sierra-leone/
[2] http://www.globalgiving.org/projects/girls-off-the-street/updates
[3] http://www.emansion.gov.lr/doc/Special_State_Delivered_July%2030.pdf
[4] http://keystoneaccountability.wordpress.com/2014/11/09/putting-citizens-at-the-heart-of-the-fight-against-ebola/
[5] http://www.ft.com/cms/s/0/35e42f78-581e-11e4-b331-00144feab7de.html#axzz3IUdltSJL
[6] http://respondingtoebola.wordpress.com/2014/11/11/ripple-effects-of-ebola/
[7] At first you might assume that it misses Liberians because they speak another language. But the algorithm has no bias towards English. Most of the chatter on wordpress turns out to be in English. Liberia and Sierra

Leone are English-speaking countries in name (though not in practice). Most of the small group of Internet users there do post in English.

[8] From *The Art of War*.

10: What is the story of the international humanitarian aid response?

Since 1988 **ActionAid** has been in Sierra Leone serving over 158,000 citizens. ActionAid provides healthcare, safe childbirth, clean water, young entrepreneur training, and lobbies for pro-poor policy change. Here is ActionAid's story (edited for brevity):

17 July 2014[1]:

Ebola outbreak in West Africa is believed to have killed more than 4,500[2] people already.

1 August 2014[3]:

Sierra Leone: people view hospitals as death zones. People who are sick [for any reason] are afraid to go for treatment in case their neighbours suspect they are carrying Ebola.

Talk of enforcing quarantines on whole villages and carrying out door to door searches, actions which effectively criminalise people for falling sick and being scared, only serves to make the problem worse.

Markets closed. Price of soap and bleach skyrocketing.

21 August 2014[4]:

Some people don't believe Ebola is a real virus. Many people are consulting traditional healers or are claiming it is caused by witchcraft.

10th September 2014[5]:

We are asking staff not involved in the Ebola response to stay at home part of the week, providing them with mobile phones and portable modems to allow them to work remotely. Our offices now have not only sanitizers and improved hand washing facilities but also infra-red thermometers to scan the temperature of visitors as they arrive.

We don't want to bring people together for meetings or workshops when it might expose people to infection.

16 October 2014[6]:

Ebola is pulling my country apart. Liberia is a nation recovering from war. A nation that has spent ten years rebuilding its broken infrastructure. Our health systems are underfunded, but our economy was recovering. Now our poor are getting poorer.

A couple of weeks ago I met a man so destitute he brought his critically ill son to an Ebola holding centre in a wheelbarrow. Wearing no protective clothing, except a thin pair of rubber gloves, he explained that his son was bleeding, that he had been vomiting and was so weak he couldn't stand.

I was horrified when the centre turned him away, because there was simply no space to admit him. We called the Ebola helpline, a national response centre where people who have symptoms of the disease are supposed to get help. But we were simply told to "be patient". They had known about the boy's case for four days.

Multinational companies are scaling down. The price of food is soaring.

The [temporarily] quarantined communities of West Point and Dolo Town were highly militarised. People were mistrustful and angry, not just of the army, but of aid workers too.

West Point is home to 78,000 people and is a major economic hub. Richer Liberians normally go there to buy fish, meat and vegetables, so the quarantine has had a crippling impact on local livelihoods.

3 November 2014[7]:

When people leave treatment centres they do not even have the clothes on their backs as everything they have touched has to be destroyed. Many people have lost everything and have no money to purchase new items. We heard that doctors and nurses had been giving their own clothes to Ebola patients, but now the demand is too great. We are giving out survivor packs to people who are discharged from the treatment centres.

Our survivor kits provide clothes and basic toiletries like toothpaste and soap as well as food - essentials that not only help people keep themselves fed and clean but also help them retain their dignity.

We also provide food and supplies for those who are put into quarantine after being in contact with someone who has Ebola - as often they have no other way of getting food.

One survivor's story:

A few weeks ago my father-in-law died from what we thought was malaria. As we are Muslims he was buried the same day. My husband and his brother took part in the burial ceremony. Five days later my mother-in-law fell ill and died and then my brother-in-law.

My husband was panicked and realised that this was not normal and said it could be Ebola. A few days later he started running a fever and asked me to take him to the Ebola treatment centre at the hospital in Monrovia. I took him and luckily for us he was accepted into the centre. Every day for nine days I made the journey from our home to the centre which took up to 2 hours and having to change taxi bus three times just to see him and check how he was.

Other members of the family did not want anything to do with me and my kids.

While we were in quarantine we got supplies of rice, oil, sanitary supplies, soap and hand washing buckets and chlorax for disinfecting. They talked to the children and encouraged me to be strong.

6 November 2014:

Not a single U.S.-promised treatment bed has been delivered to the country. However, the first treatment center built by the US government did open 4 days later.

As the rainy season is ending in West Africa, experts fear that travel between affected countries might increase and that the virus could reenter areas previously thought to be Ebola-free.

10 November 2014[8]:

In Ebola affected Sierra Leone, Liberia and Guinea, one in seven women could die in childbirth.

Last week I saw a woman who was forced to give birth on her own because everyone around her - even the nurses - were too scared to touch her, in case she had Ebola. Luckily she gave birth to a healthy baby girl, who she named 'Miracle'.

Doctors without Borders (known elsewhere as "Medecins sans Frontiers" in French, or MSF) has been responding to the West Africa Ebola outbreak since March 2014. As of November 2014, MSF had 3,340 staff working in Guinea, Liberia and Sierra Leone, treating a rapidly increasing number of patients. This are some milestones from their worker blogs and operational updates:

24 July 2014[9]:

In the past three weeks, MSF has trained more than 200 community health workers to deliver essential health messages to people in their villages about how to protect themselves against Ebola and what action to take if someone shows any signs or symptoms of the disease.

Guinea: MSF closed its Ebola treatment centre in Telimélé after no new cases were reported for 21 days.

8 August 2014[10,11]:

The situation in the Liberian capital, Monrovia, is "catastrophic," with over 40 health workers recently infected.

MSF currently has 66 international and 610 national staff responding to the crisis in the three affected countries. All our Ebola experts are mobilized, we simply cannot do more.

15 August 2014[12]:

We are seeing a totally different scenario than what we have seen in past. It is an open epidemic, reaching urban areas and not isolated to a few villages. It is destroying the healthcare system in Liberia and Sierra Leone. Without basic healthcare, we are likely to see deaths from common illnesses such as malaria and diarrhoea.

Kailahun, Sierra Leone: we urgently need to follow up 2,000 people who came into contact with Ebola patients, but we can only follow up with 200 of them, given our staff size.

We hear of deaths of many more people than we have the capacity to verify.

Foya, Liberia: We had 137 patients at 40-bed Ebola treatment centre. Our laboratory has a backlog of tests to run on suspected cases. In Monrovia we started created a 120-bed facility, but MSF has never managed a care center of this size before.

5 September 2014[13]:

Before contracting the disease, Eric had been working as head nurse in the Ebola Case Management Centre (CMC). They took his body home to the small village of Yassadou of around 300 people, hidden in the forested highlands of northern Liberia, for burial.

The entire village appears. Upset, screaming, and sobbing, some run around with their arms in the air. Some drop to the floor and writhe in the dust. These images are burned in my brain. The parish priest begins to pray: "God, may you help us to understand the concept of this terrible disease. We cannot do much for Eric anymore. He is in your arms now. May Eric rest in peace. Amen." He then turns to the residents of Yassadou: "What you can do now is protect yourself. Let's believe that Ebola is real."

Before the burial starts an MSF health worker explains, "So much wrong information is spreading around in Liberia. Ebola is not airborne transmitted and salty water or oil cannot prevent you from it. We don't know where these false messages are coming from, but please stop believing them."

Women start chanting while MSF hygienists take Eric's coffin out of the car. One member of staff ceaselessly sprays chlorine solution on the caretakers, their gloves and their boots. Nearby men stare at the MSF burial team in their yellow plastic bodysuits, gloves and facial masks. Some are covering their mouths to protect themselves from the smell.

As the coffin is put slowly into the freshly dug earth, raindrops pour down. Eric's brother Johnson-Boie grabs a shovel and silently covers his brother's grave with wet earth.

12 September 2014[14]:

Soon after arriving in Monrovia, I realised that my colleagues were overwhelmed by the scale of the Ebola outbreak. Our treatment centre - the biggest MSF has ever run - was full. It was my job to stand at the gate and turn people away.

For the first three days that I stood at the gate it rained hard. People were drenched, but they carried on waiting because they had nowhere else to go.

The first person I had to turn away was a father who had brought his sick daughter in the trunk of his car. He was an educated man, and he pleaded with me to take his teenage daughter, saying that whilst he knew we couldn't save her life, at least we could save the rest of his family from her. At that point I had to go behind one of the tents to cry.

Other families just pulled up in cars, let the sick person out and then drove off, abandoning them. One mother tried to leave her baby on a chair, hoping that if she did, we would have no choice but to care for the child.

I had to turn away one couple who arrived with their young daughter. Two hours later the girl died in front of our gate, where she remained until the body removal team took her away.

There was no way of letting more patients in without putting everyone, and all of our work, at risk.

One afternoon a nurse came to find me, saying there was something I had to see. Whenever people recover and are discharged, we hold a small celebration with them. Hearing the words of the discharged patients as they thank us for what we did, gives us all a good reason to be there. The nurse turned to me and said, "Thank you. I could never do the work that you do, out there at the front gate."

25 September 2014[15,16]:

MSF now operates six treatment centres providing 549 additional hospital beds in the region, [effectively doubling the capacity of the healthcare system]. We admitted 3,299 patients, diagnosed 2,051 cases of Ebola, and 650 have survived. This cost about 50 million dollars. An example of the value of this work follows with this Ebola survivor's story:

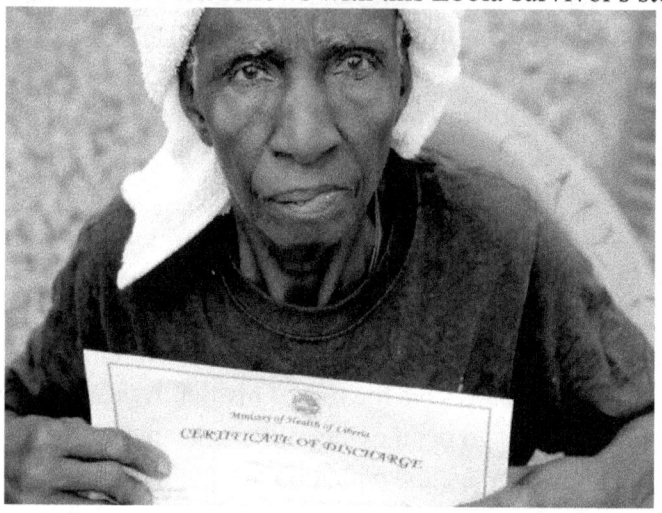

The elderly lady with her sweet-tempered eyes has worked all her life in rice fields. Until now she had avoided taking any medication in her life. Nessie was found in her house with all the symptoms of Ebola - diarrhoea, fever, nausea, headache and body aches, red eyes and hiccups.

She was brought to the CMC, and for more than two hours she had to endure a trip on roads that do not even deserve a name, only to be received by the doctors shaking their heads. No one gave her a glimmer of hope for survival.

Right up until the end of her stay, nobody could convince her that she had been infected with Ebola. "It must have been the flu," she says with a tender smile. However, she is delighted about her certificate of discharge, as it hopefully prevents bad gossip from her neighbours. In these times, Ebola is closely followed by its evil twin brother called stigma. Many Ebola survivors have to cope with it after their recovery. What an exceptional immune system this woman 90+ year old woman must have!

21 October 2014[17]:

I was out working with MSF as a health promotion officer, visiting villages and telling people about Ebola: how to protect themselves and their families, what to do if they start to develop symptoms, and making sure everyone has the MSF hotline number to call.

My wife did not believe in Ebola. I called her, begging her to leave Monrovia and bring the children north so we could be together here. She did not listen. She denied Ebola.

Late one night, my brother called me. 'Your wife has died.' I said, 'what?' He said, 'Bendu is dead.' I dropped the phone. I threw it away and it broke apart. We were together for 23 years. She understood me. She was the only one who understood me very well. I felt like I'd lost my whole memory. My eyes were open, but I didn't know what I was looking at. I had no vision.

Later I learned that my brother, who was working as a nurse, had been taking care of my wife and had become infected too. Then my two youngest children were taken to the centre in Monrovia. My girls were very sick and they died. I felt even more helpless. I was breaking in my mind. I couldn't make sense of anything.

My eldest son, Kollie James, was still in Monrovia in the house where our family had been sick, though he was showing no signs of illness. He called me and said, 'everyone got sick, I don't know what to do.' I told him to come here to Foya to be with me.

When my son arrived, people in the village would not accept us. They told us that our family had all died and to take Kollie James away. I was angered by their reaction. I knew he wasn't showing any symptoms and was not a threat to them but because of the stigma, they wouldn't let us stay.

The next morning, though I noticed my son looking more tired than usual. I called the Ebola hotline and MSF brought him to their Ebola care centre here in Foya to be tested. When the test came back positive, it was a night of agony for me.

Every day, the counselors made sure they saw me, and they sat with me so I could talk.

Then MSF told me, that Kollie is the 1000th survivor from Ebola. Now that my son is free of Ebola we will make a life for ourselves.

30 October 2014[18]:

The global response to Ebola must be structured and coherent; however it is scattered and piecemeal. MSF is still the only organisation operating new treatment centers.

In Monrovia there were around 80 patients in the 250-bed facility. MSF teams are looking into the reasons for the sudden drop in patients coming in. We speculate that a widespread aversion to the government's mandatory cremation policy, poor ambulance service, poor referral systems, and changes in behaviour may explain the drop. Patient numbers could go up again.

We have distributed 44,154 Ebola kits in Monrovia alone. These kits help families treat people with symptoms and safely handle people who have died at home. They are in no way meant as a substitute for the care provided our CMCs. MSF also aims to reach 300,000 people with anti-malaria treatment to avoid the need for people to come into the already overcrowded hospitals.

In Sierra Leone, the government has put five of the worst affected districts under quarantine. Roadblocks affect one to two million people. There is minimal surveillance as 85 percent of telephone calls to the national Ebola hotline go unanswered.

5 November, 2014[19]:

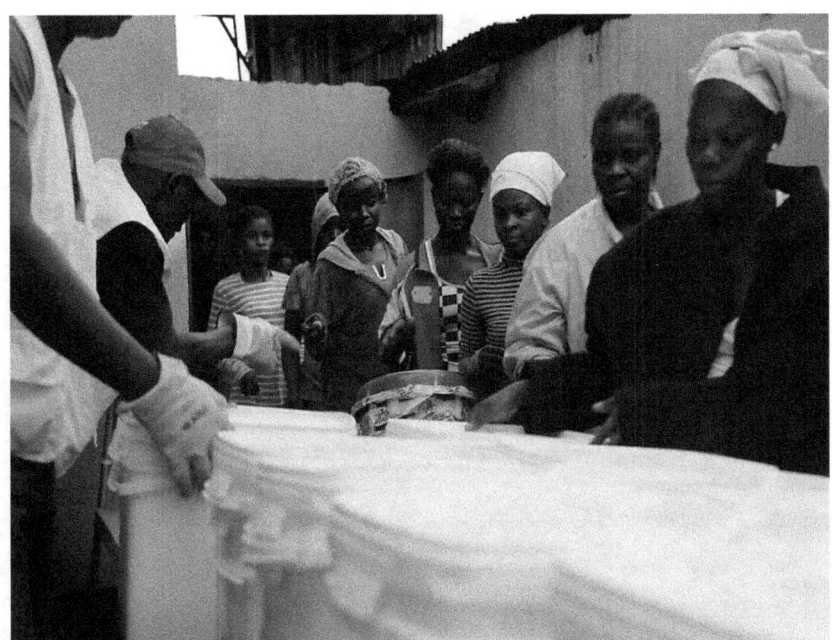

Ebola home kits: The buckets are put on a table and people come to pick them up in groups of ten. The team set up a circuit: people enter from a football pitch, form a queue, pick up their kits and exit onto the street. "It is a very physical job," says Emmanuel. "You need to do everything in one go: give the kits, communicate with people and ask them to move fast."

An imperfect solution for disinfecting their home after a family member dies.

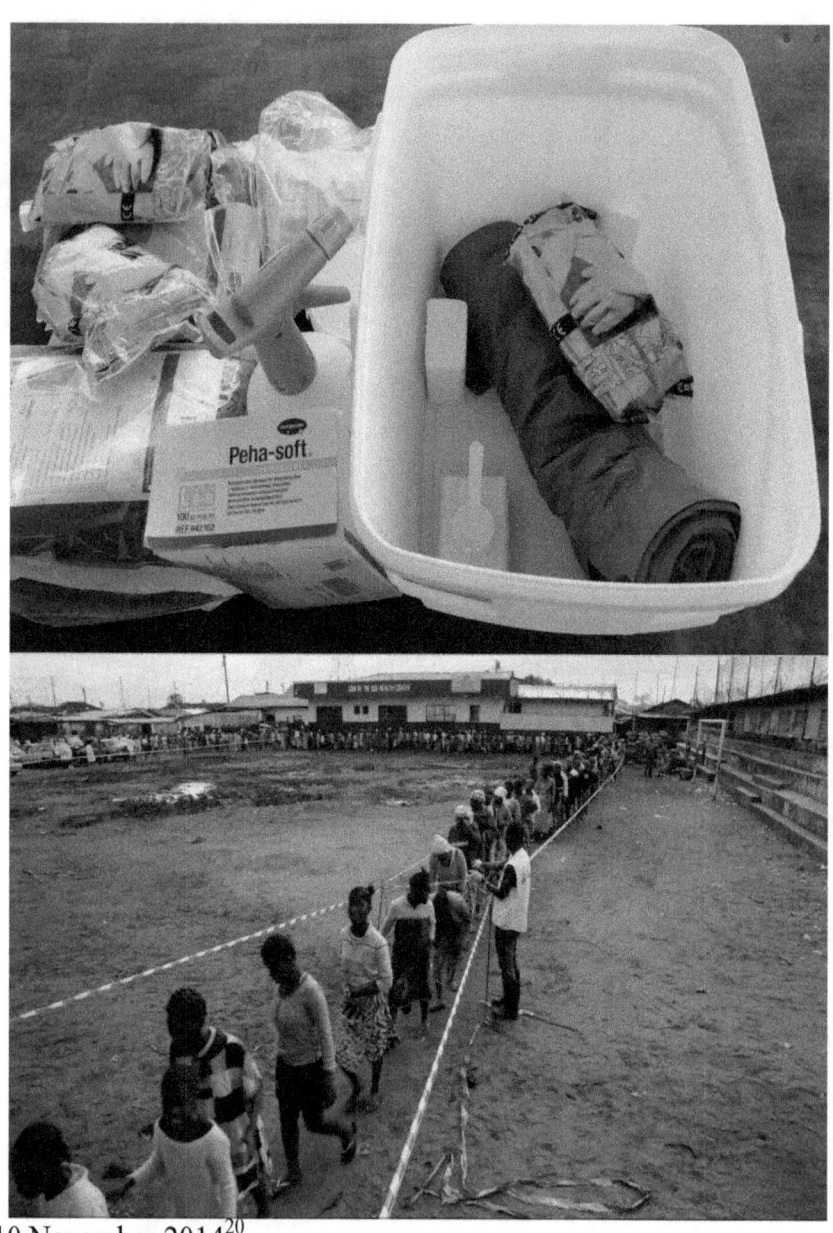

10 November 2014[20]:

While cases in Liberia in decline, cases in Guinea and Sierra Leone are on the rise.

The Liberian healthcare system has virtually collapsed because of the epidemic. Many hospitals and clinics are closed, and those that are running turn feverish or vomiting patients away for fear they have Ebola.

Much of the international aid funding for the Ebola response is earmarked for specific projects. Instead, international donors and implementing organisations should deploy their resources with flexibility so that they can be used where they are needed most.

11 November 2014:

Statement from Craig Spencer, MSF volunteer that contracted Ebola and was evacuated to New York for treatment, and later released:

"For over five weeks, I worked in an Ebola treatment center in Guéckédou, the epicenter of the outbreak. During this time, I cried as I held children who were not strong enough to survive the virus. But, I also experienced immense joy when patients I treated were cured and invited me into their family as a brother upon discharge. Within a week of my diagnosis, many of these same patients called my personal phone to wish me well and ask if there was any way they could contribute to my care. Most incredibly, I watched my Guinean colleagues, who have been on the front lines since day one and saw friends and family members die, continue to fight to save their communities with so much compassion and dignity. They are the heroes that we are not talking about."

Over the same timeframe, the **World Health Organization** provided regular "situation updates" with a lot of dry facts. These are the few personal notes that stand out from the lot, pulled from http://www.who.int/mediacentre/news/ebola/en/:

15 August 2014[21]:

One source of public misunderstanding, especially in the affected areas, comes from rumors on social media claiming that certain products or practices can prevent or cure Ebola virus disease. In Nigeria, for example, at least two people have died after drinking salt water, rumored to be protective.

22 August 2014[22]:

The scope of the outbreak is underestimated. Many deny that a patient has Ebola and believe that care in an isolation ward - viewed as an incubator of the disease - will lead to infection and certain death. In rural villages, corpses are buried without notifying health officials and with no investigation of the cause of death. Fresh graves are often the only crude indicator to estimate the number of new cases.

As soon as a new treatment facility is opened, it is immediately filled with patients, many of whom were not previously identified.

8 September 2014[23]:

In Montserrado county (Monrovia), the team estimated that 1000 beds are urgently needed for the treatment of currently infected Ebola patients. At present only 240 beds are available, with an additional 260 beds either planned or in the process of being put in place.

The John F Kennedy Medical Center in Monrovia, which was largely destroyed during Liberia's civil war, remains the country's only academic referral hospital. The hospital is plagued by electrical fires and floods, and several medical staff were infected there and died, depleting the hospital's limited workforce further.

West Point slum in Monrovia, which has no sanitation, little running water, and virtually no electrical supplies is a major concern.

Conventional Ebola control interventions are not having an adequate impact in Liberia. Far greater community engagement is the cornerstone of a more effective response. Where communities have taken charge and created their own solutions and protective measures, Ebola transmission has slowed considerably.

26 September 2014[24]:

Never before in recorded history has a biosafety level four pathogen infected so many people so quickly, over such a broad geographical area, for so long.

6 November 2014[25]:

The first clinical trials of therapeutic - possibly curative - transfusions of whole blood or blood plasma from recovered patients are scheduled to begin soon in Liberia, in line with WHO technical guidelines.

In another study, patients older than 40 years were nearly 3.5 times more likely to die than those aged less than 40.

The United States Government through its military, the Center for Disease Control, USAID, and the state department promised a lot of action. These milestones show that it is far less agile and capable of meeting the timeframe that countering this kind of epidemic requires that MSF. In the time it has taken these government agencies to set a course of action, MSF was able to effectively double the healthcare capacity of the region. It was putting down a new hospital every 4 weeks, and doing it at far less cost. Moreover, two thirds of the MSF effort was funded by regular people making small direct donations. Here is the US government's timeline, based on Voice of America announcements in the region:

4 August 2014[26]:

"The U.S. Centers for Disease Control is sending 50 public health experts to help three West African nations battling Ebola." This statement was tagged onto the end of most VOA news stories for more than a week.

22 September 2014[27]:

About 60 military personnel arrived in West Africa as part of the U.S. effort to combat Ebola. The United States has committed $175 million to help combat the outbreak and is sending 3,000 troops to the region to build more than a dozen 100-bed field hospitals.

25 September 2014[28]:

The president announced last week a $1 billion-plus U.S. plan to help West African nations contain Ebola. Meanwhile, the World Bank says it is giving another $170 million to the West African nations hardest hit by the disease to help them contain its spread, adding to the $230 million it had already approved.

28 October 2014[29]:

"The world's response has been late and incomplete. This is a tragedy at many, many levels. And obviously people are dying, commerce is impacted, economic development is impacted, but, overwhelmingly, people are dying and we could have done a better job as a global community. There have been some groups that have been absolutely fantastic like Doctors Without Borders and individual aid groups have been putting their own lives at stake. But the global community has dropped the ball," said Dr. Harvey Rubin in New Scientist Magazine. Rubin is director of the Institute for Strategic Threat Analysis and Response.

29 October 2014[30]:

U.S. Ambassador to the United Nations Samantha Power has promised a sustained response to the West African Ebola crisis.

Also Thursday, the World Bank pledged $100 million to help recruit more foreign health care workers to treat Ebola patients in West Africa, along with $400 million already sent.

10 November 2014:

The first Ebola treatment center built and staffed by the US government opens in Liberia. About 2100 US government and army workers are now operating in the region.[31]

14 November 2014:

The head of USAID called on Congress to approve President Obama's pending request for $6.2 billion in emergency funding to combat the deadly disease. Vice President Joe Biden praised religious groups for helping fight Ebola by promoting safe burial practices, which sometimes clash with religious tradition. Local traditions in West Africa have rapidly changed to curb the number of cases stemming from handling corpses during burial rites.

[1] http://www.actionaid.org.uk/news-and-views/news-blog/2014/07/17/the-race-to-contain-ebola-photos-from-the-frontline-of-an?slide=2

[2] This is a much higher estimate than the official counts were giving in July. Action Aid gave no source on their blog post. But I personally think we will learn later that the true number of deaths is much higher than the official count, because the public was afraid to visit hospitals for months before it attracted international attention.

[3] http://www.actionaid.org.uk/news-and-views/news-blog/2014/08/01/fighting-the-ebola-outbreak-on-the-ground

[4] http://www.actionaid.org.uk/news-and-views/news-blog/2014/08/21/ebola-outbreak-whats-the-latest

[5] http://www.actionaid.org.uk/news-and-views/news-blog/2014/09/10/keeping-staff-safe-while-ebola-spreads-like-wildfire

[6] http://www.actionaid.org.uk/about-us/voices-blog/2014/10/16/ebola-is-pulling-my-country-apart-a-letter-from-liberia

[7] http://www.actionaid.org.uk/about-us/voices-blog/2014/11/03/helping-the-people-left-behind-when-someone-dies-of-ebola

[8] http://www.actionaid.org.uk/news-and-views/news-blog/2014/11/10/giving-birth-in-an-ebola-epidemic-1-in-7-women-could-die

[9] http://www.msf.org/article/operational-update-ebola-outbreak-west-africa

[10] http://www.msf.org/article/msf-operational-update-ebola-outbreak-west-africa

[11] http://www.msf.org/article/ebola-official-msf-response-who-declaring-ebola-international-public-health-emergency

[12] http://www.msf.org/article/new-strategies-and-more-hands-capacity-needed-curb-ebola-epidemic

[13] http://www.msf.org/article/ebola-erics-last-walk

[14] http://www.msf.org/article/liberia-somebody-had-do-it-turning-people-away-overwhelmed-ebola-treatment-centre

[15] http://blogs.msf.org/en/staff/blogs/msf-ebola-blog/miracles-happen

[16] http://www.msf.org/article/ebola-crisis-update-sept-25th

[17] http://www.msf.org/article/my-son-msf%E2%80%99s-1000th-ebola-survivor

[18] http://www.msf.org/article/ebola-crisis-update-30th-october-2014

[19] http://www.msf.org/article/liberia-distributing-home-disinfection-kits-west-point-suburb

[20] http://www.msf.org/article/ebola-hard-won-gains-liberia-must-not-be-undermined

[21] http://www.who.int/mediacentre/news/ebola/15-august-2014/en/

[22] http://www.who.int/mediacentre/news/ebola/22-august-2014/en/

[23] http://www.who.int/mediacentre/news/ebola/8-september-2014/en/

[24] http://www.who.int/mediacentre/news/ebola/26-september-2014/en/

[25] http://www.who.int/mediacentre/news/ebola/06-november-2014/en/

[26] http://www.voanews.com/content/nigeria-reports-second-ebola-case/1971091.html

[27] http://www.voanews.com/content/sierra-leone-ends-ebola-lockdown-expects-rise-in-cases/2457797.html

[28] http://www.voanews.com/content/obama-to-address-un-ebola-meeting/2462000.html

[29] http://www.voanews.com/content/infectious-disease-new-response-28oct14/2499320.html

[30] http://www.voanews.com/content/us-diplomat-promises-sustained-response-to-ebola-outbreak/2500934.html

[31] http://www.usaid.gov/news-information/press-releases/nov-10-2014-first-us-constructed-ebola-treatment-unit-set-open-liberia

11: Who is trying to profit from Ebola and how?

When asked the open-ended question in a Gallup poll, "what are the biggest problems facing the country?" one in 20 Americans cited Ebola (5%). The economy (17%) and dissatisfaction with government (16%) were the top two concerns.[1] In another poll, two thirds of Americans believed Ebola would become an epidemic in the United States, compared to one third who thought the government was doing all it could. In the same Washington Post poll, third thirds of Americans favored a travel ban on West Africans coming into America[2]. A poll from the conservative newspaper *The Washington Times* found that 93 percent of readers favored the ban. People are alarmed.

Fear is one of the most powerful emotional triggers, and marketers know that. They usually have a limited set of tools to make people buy whatever they're selling. One list from a marketer gives just seven triggers: lust, mystique, alarm, prestige, power, vice, and trust.[3] The threat of Ebola evokes so much terror, alarm, and fear that the less scrupulous bunch inevitably can't resist exploit public fears. The fact that these fears are totally irrational and unfounded even assuages their guilt a little.

Some exploits are obvious. Ebolasuits.com popped up to sell hazmat suits to anyone who wants one. They're happy to let you decide how much money you can give them to feel safe, ranging from the very modestly priced "original Ebola suit" at $34.99 to the "long-term survival suit" at $1,499.00 - essentially a space suit. The website's developer carefully wove the fear of Ebola with distrust of the government in his comment to ThinkProgress.org, saying, "If this thing does get big, you can't depend on the federal government to distribute suits.[4]" He knows his target audience worries about both things.

Legitimate medical suppliers have gotten in on the action too. After noting tons of traffic to their site from people searching for "Ebola kits," sellers Mountainside Medical Equipment and Outpatient-MD repackaged a first aid kit into a new product, an "Ebola kit" and saw sales go up.[5] This is an ethical "gray area" -

marking to demand - because at least the product offers protection against Ebola, should a person ever need to be protected in the future (a very very remote possibility in USA for the foreseeable future). Much worse are people who are sell a product that offers no protection, because it is based on a popular misperception about Ebola. Someone kept bringing air filters up on our reddit AMA. He asked the team in West Africa why they weren't using high tech air filters. Response: "Because Ebola is not airborne." Restating the facts often won't stop people from buying as many "just in case" solutions as they can afford. The entire "prepper" industry is based on exploiting humans' irrational fear of gruesome but improbable scenarios. Humans are quite poor at comparing the relative risk of two remote possibilities. Are you more likely to die from a shark attack[6], a lightning strike[7], or falling off a ladder while at work?[8] Answer: (75 vs 43 vs 115) Ladders are 50% more dangerous than sharks and three times as dangerous as lightning! But if you shouldn't believe that either. Instead, you should realize that all of these threats are negligible. There is a near-zero probability that you will die from any of these causes, even though 15,460 people fell off ladders last year alone. Less than 1% of people who fall off a ladder die, and the number who climb ladders and actually fall is a number so small I'd need to use scientific notation just to write it. What you should be worrying about are heart disease, cancer, and diabetes - all preventable, and far more likely to affect your life if you don't exercise and eat well. Once again, a misunderstanding of science is enabling people to profit. Conspiracy theorists have been looking for evidence to prove that Ebola is a hoax, much like they did with HIV/AIDS in the 1980s[9]. Upon deeper inspection, they misinterpreted each line of evidence.

"This is not Ebola."[10]

One blogger wrote:
There is something missing in this Ebola outbreak, and it is the bloody eyes and ears, and bleeding through the skin. All

the bloody blistered skin photos on the web are from previous outbreaks, with this particular strain people look outwardly normal up until death and die from internal bleeding, vomiting up blood and having massive stools of black goo from internal bleeding.

He also claimed that the virus is mutating too rapidly to be Ebola. This is not true. All viruses mutate rapidly and there is no such thing as a "stable virus." Viruses have no cellular machinery of their own, and hence have no means of controlling their own mutation rate the way that bacteria and humans do. Moreover, Ebola only infected a few hundred people from 1976 to 2014, so the "wild" mutation rate would have been difficult to measure.

Nothing is "missing" in this epidemic. The symptoms he is looking for were originally exaggerated in the best-selling virus scare book, *The Hot Zone*. Even its author Richard Preston admits to exaggerating his description of the disease in an interview:[11]

> Eyes can turn brilliant red from blood vessels leaking and blood oozing out of the eyelid. In the original *Hot Zone*, I have a description of a nurse 'weeping tears of blood.' But that almost certainly didn't happen.

A commentary on *Hot Zone* from Tara Smith in Science Magazine adds:[12]

> Over and over, he uses words like "dissolving," "liquefy," "bleeding out" to describe patient pathology. (If I had been playing a drinking game while reading and did a shot every time Preston uses "liquefy" in the book, I'd be dead right now).

Tara provides an excerpt from the book to illustrate:

> He coughs a deep cough and regurgitates something into the bag. The bag swells up…. you see that his lips are smeared with something slippery and red, mixed with black specks, as if he has been chewing coffee grounds. His eyes are the color of rubies, and his face is an expressionless mask of bruises. The red spots… have expanded and merged into huge,

spontaneous purple shadows; his whole head is turning black-and-blue.... The connective tissue of his face is dissolving, and his face appears to hang from the underlying bone, as if the face is detaching itself from the skull.

Tara writes:

Local stories are scary enough when the reality of the virus is exposed, and with it the dual affliction of poverty and the terrible health system.

She quotes a spokesperson for MSF, who provides a more accurate description:

The patients mostly look sick and weak. If there is blood, it is not a lot, usually in the vomit or diarrhea, occasionally from the gums or nose.

Preston has a talent for creative and dramatic interpretations of events that grab the public on a primal level. In 2014 he plans to inject a new metaphor into a rewrite of his book (from the same interview):

With the science that we have now, we can perceive Ebola as being not one thing but as a swarm, and the swarm is moving through the human population and expanding its numbers. It has the qualities of a monster.

It is no wonder that people in search of conspiracy theories have latched on to his version of Ebola as evidence that the real outbreak must be something else. Preston's description is closer to the face melting scene in *Raiders of the Lost Ark*. No disease could live up to that hype. It is a good thing Tara Smith and *Science Magazine* are aggressively trying to correct the record. We must all choose a balance between injecting drama into events to grab readers attention, and creating a fantasy plague that will cause people to overreact to a threat.

To his credit, Preston also tried to quash some of the lies that others used his book to propagate. In that interview he said:

We know a lot more about Ebola in the intervening 20 years. Initially, there were a lot of fears that Ebola could mutate to become the airborne Andromeda strain that would wipe us all out. Ebola does not travel through the air in airborne form and is very unlikely to mutate that way. Another thing that's been learned about Ebola is the mutation rate. The virus is continually mutating as it's moving through the human population. It's testing out its new environment. One of the biggest concerns is that all of our drugs and tests and vaccines for Ebola need to be adjusted. We can adjust the tests, but we need to watch how the virus is mutating.

That nuance has been misunderstood by bloggers predicting that "**any new Ebola vaccine will be worthless.**" The rationale is that it will keep mutating faster than we can create vaccines to stop it. This is true, but it also true for all diseases. We continue to create new antibiotics to replace those that are no longer effective. Bacteria continuously mutate (some would say "evolve"). Mutant strains eventually yield resistant strains. The more we overmedicate the population, the stronger the selection pressure on bacteria to evolve becomes. So it is natural and unavoidable that any vaccine may be rendered useless at some point. What is misleading is to claim that the vaccine will be useless as soon as it is produced. The worst-case scenario is that Ebola mutates so quickly and so effectively are vaccines are rendered useless every year, like the flu virus. There is evidence that this is not likely to happen. Ebola mutates in a random way, and 99.999% of mutations make Ebola less dangerous. It's the 0.001% that pose a threat, but not an overnight threat.

The Ebola vaccine conspiracy is wrapped up in a larger conspiracy against all vaccines that is utterly wrong. Here is a list of facts that this paranoid lot use to construct their arguments:[13]
1. Vaccines don't work.
2. Vaccines cause the very diseases they are alleged to prevent.
3. Vaccines are full of dangerous toxins.
4. The UK government and the vaccine industry colluded to hide these facts from the public so they would continue to take vaccines.

5. The UK government and the vaccine industry colluded to prevent safety studies.

These are half-truths. There are examples of vaccines that *no longer* work, and ones that did not work, but all the currently required vaccines do work. Diseases much worse than Ebola have been eradicated because of vaccines. Vaccines do cause the disease in rare cases - less than one in a million. We know of no other way to train a person's immune system to recognize a pathogen other than injecting a tiny dose of that pathogen into the body. That's how immunity is conferred.

Some vaccines have at some point in the past contained a preservative that was considered harmful, and later removed. To ship a vaccine without preservatives would ensure that many people were injected with something that no longer conferred immunity, or with some dangerous pathogen growing in the syringe. All preservatives currently appear safe. Preservatives make it possible to deliver vaccines to most of the world, where refrigeration is still a rarity. And about the collusion - the bulk of the 45-page report is about the government's poor track record at responding to questions of whether vaccines were entirely safe for children. You can read and decide for yourself, but I think the evidence falls far short of collusion.

"Ebola is a bioweapon created by the US army in a lab."

This is the implicit assumption behind a whole collection of conspiracies. There is the supposed "smoking gun" document - a 2009 wikileaks cable that proves the **US Army withheld promise from Germany that Ebola virus wouldn't be weaponized**[14]. The actual substance of this disagreement is a missing rubber stamp on the document. Part of the memo reads: "The enclosed end use certificate is on the letterhead of the U.S. Army. The required official seal is missing."[15] Nothing in the source document implies any discussion about or intent to weaponize Ebola.

Another blog, typical of this flavor of conspiracy, lists every news report over the last twenty years about accidents in biolabs or official comments about bioweapons.[16] What is significantly absent from this list is anything from after 2012. Given the hours the author must have spent highlighting in bold all the scary words in these quotes, I assume he searched for recent reports and didn't find any. It relies on a logical fallacy: Because "accidents have occurred" in bio labs and the US government has created bioweapons in labs, they hope the reader will assume that this outbreak must therefore be caused by an accident in a bioweapons facility. If you want a comprehensive history of every person who ever got infected with Ebola in a research lab, David Quammen's book, *Ebola: The natural and human history of a deadly virus*[17] offers the best digest. Whatever the government's intent was in the past, there are far better pathogens to use as a bio-weapon.

Some other ridiculous conspiracies about Ebola circulated the around the Internet recently:

- "Ebola is caused by chem trails - poison and dangerous - hold your breath - sickness from the sky."
- Global elites bioengineered Ebola in order to impose quarantines, travel bans and eventually martial law on the planet.
- Or they created it for global population control.
- CDC patented the virus and to make a fortune from a new vaccine it had created with the pharmaceutical industry.

Context: CDC did patent a strain of Ebola in 2010, but this happens with other CDC work too. Government patents are an important way to prevent for-profit companies from claiming sole-ownership of genetic code, as one company tried to do with the human genome project in the 1990s.

All of these conspiracies reveal who we are to ourselves: We are distrustful of government, its agencies, and corporations to have our best interests in mind.

---

[1] http://www.gallup.com/poll/178742/ebola-debuts-americans-list-top-problems.aspx

[2] http://www.washingtonpost.com/national/health-science/ebola-poll-two-thirds-of-americans-worried-about-possible-widespread-epidemic-in-us/2014/10/13/d0afd0ee-52ff-11e4-809b-8cc0a295c773_story.html

[3] http://ebscolearning.com/2014/08/22/fascinate-your-7-triggers-to-persuasion-and-captivation/

[4] http://thinkprogress.org/health/2014/10/17/3581209/ebola-fears-spawn-profit/

[5] http://thinkprogress.org/health/2014/10/17/3581209/ebola-fears-spawn-profit/

[6] http://en.wikipedia.org/wiki/Shark_attack

[7] http://www.lightningsafety.noaa.gov/fatalities.htm

[8] http://ehstoday.com/construction/cdc-there-s-nothing-easy-about-falling-ladder

[9] http://www.aidstruth.org/denialism/myths

[10] http://www.jimstonefreelance.com/ebolanotnormal.html

[11] http://www.nytimes.com/2014/10/20/books/the-hot-zone-author-tracks-ebolas-evolution.html?_r=1

[12] http://scienceblogs.com/aetiology/2014/10/21/the-hot-zone-and-the-mythos-of-ebola/

[13] http://exopolitics.blogs.com/ebolagate/2014/10/will-ebola-vaccines-be-safe-and-effective-what-foia-documents-in-the-uk-and-us-reveal.html cited this as its primary source: https://childhealthsafety.wordpress.com/2012/03/14/government-experts-cover-up-vaccine-hazards/ cited this as its primary source: http://nsnbc.me/wp-content/uploads/2013/05/BSEM-2011.pdf

[14] http://rt.com/news/197500-us-army-ebola-weapon/

[15] https://wikileaks.org/plusd/cables/09BERLIN1588_a.html#efmAYPAhB

[16] http://www.washingtonsblog.com/2014/10/ebola-2.html

[17] http://www.amazon.com/Ebola-Natural-Human-History-Deadly/dp/0393351556

12: Ebola: There's an app for that?

For as long as we've had cell phones, people have been promising an economic renaissance in Africa shouldered by technology. When I was in the Peace Corps in Gambia (1999), the Internet was "destined" to bring limitless knowledge to a generation of school children. Instead, every one of the dozen schools I worked with had broken Internet for eleven months out of the year, because they couldn't pay the phone bill.[1] And when I studied how Internet was being used in West Africa as a Fulbright in 2003-2004, I found that a mix of email ("pen friends!"), chat, and instant messenger were what drove teens to the Internet café. Virtually no one was using the Internet to access knowledge or train for a better job. That didn't stop UN Secretary General Kofi Annan from anointing technology the savior of Africa in his speeches.

So I come to the world of solving problems with smart phone apps a bit of a skeptic. In my two years living in Kenya (2011-2013) I visited the iHUB - an incubator for tech start ups - weekly and followed a dozen entrepreneurs try to launch the "next big thing." I witnessed the World Bank pitch their open data platform there, extolling the wonders of "free data" to a group of Kenyan app developers. The celebration was over when the first developer raised an unsteady hand and asked the right question:

> With all this data… say I build an app and some citizen uses it. Say he learns the local government is stealing from you… where is the email address or phone number of the person in the World Bank that he can call to report corruption about a specific project?

The speaker waffled, made some vague promises to follow-up, and was quickly forgotten. Since then, no apps have emerged there using that data. It lacked something crucial; it was about things, not people.

The only kind of technology that has actually made a difference in Africa is the kind built around relationships. Demand for email, chat, and the latest messaging services (currently whatsApp) is what's behind the ridiculous number of cell phones sold there. There are more cell phones than people in use in Africa today. Facebook joined the mix (Did they fear losing the market to a competitor?) when they launched Facebook Zero[2]. In the 40 poorest countries, Facebook pays the phone company for any data charges its users rack up, making it essentially the only free website on the Internet for over 500 million of the world's poor. To them, relationships are the only thing they see on the Internet. Whereas the renaissance may have made the pen mightier than the sword, smart phones are making the friends list mightier than the spreadsheet. This rule extends to the latest apps being build to fight Ebola.

Last week (early November 2014) over a thousand new smart phones showed up in our GlobalGiving office. It was the first time we'd ever accepted a "gift in kind" - a non-cash donation. There was a compelling reason - a developer named JourneyApps had interviewed first responders in Liberia and Sierra Leone and built an app to coordinate their efforts. The Android app, called "Ebola Care"[3] manages a few common tasks that NGOs and hospitals were doing by hand:

    1 - Daily checkups: Who did you meet, and what did they say?

2 - ETU transfer: You realize a child needs to be admitted to an Ebola unit. What vital details need to follow him or her?

3 - Patient Discharge: An Ebola survivor is ready to be released from quarantine, and they need a certificate and some planned follow-up.

4 - Orphans: A child's parents die and suddenly the are a ton of decisions that have to be made to manage the kid's well-being.

The app organizes all these messy tasks into categories meant to replace the tedious computer data entry that was happening before:

Contact Tracing
Finding everyone who came in direct contact with a sick Ebola patient.

Tracking orphans
Care for children abandoned due to parents contracting Ebola.

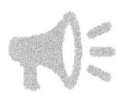

Ebola Education
Coordinate and track Ebola education events in communities.

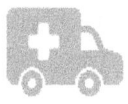

Ambulance pickups
Patient data collection by ambulance teams.

HOPE 21

HOPE 21
Observe and evaluate children under quarantine

Even though the app uses the Internet to synchronize data and share it across organizations, it doesn't require it. If a worker leaves the road she can still save data and upload it later. This is pretty complicated stuff. I know several other mobile survey platforms that spent years trying to get that one feature to work right, and chances are there will be hiccups. The company built this app in just one week. To get a minimum viable version of the app to people on the ground quickly, they simplified the problem in other ways. Everybody will be working off the same exact survey on the same model of phone, an Amazon Fire Phone. This is less likely to break than having dozens of surveys being collected on dozens of different models of phone in different languages.

GlobalGiving was the logical partner to launch it. Normally we could never get all the organizations in a region to start using the same tool, but given the severity of the crisis, they are begging us to team up. As soon as they get the phones preloaded with software their workers should be able to manage more cases in less time.

The app is by no means done, and will likely undergo a dozen revisions or more. This is at the core of good agile, management. Start up companies do the same thing if they want to survive - they launch the smallest version of a big idea that will have value for their customers and iterate on the product until it really meets a need. The philosophy is called "Lean" if you are in business, or "Agile" if you are a software company, or "Research" if you're a scientist (This idea has been around a long time but only recently is getting recognized in the non-science world).

The easy part has always been putting technology in someone's hand. The much harder part, once again, is "behavior change." In this context, two new things have to start happening: People need to enter data, and leaders need to look at the data before making a decision. Neither of these were happening before the outbreak at the level of sophistication needed to stop the disease.

An early critic of this Ebola Care App posted his complaints on UNICEFstories.org[4]. The problem with this kind of an app, he argues, is that people are doing all the work; the app isn't "smart." And by extension, the laborious task of using the app will limit people's use.

It should make life easier for nurses, health workers, and others. There is a big problem with lack of information - and lack of data - but you don't get that by distributing hardware, by itself. You get data, and information, by working with what people are already doing, and making it better. Facebook knows this - that's why it knows more about you than you know about yourself - because it's made things you want to do easier - and every time you click it gets smarter. But it's made your life easier, it's made a complicated task more simple, and it gathers information from that to understand the world. It hasn't asked you to fill out a complex survey on everything that you're interested in - Facebook knows that doing that would lose your interest, and lead to much less useful information.

Despite the app's dumbness, Imani House used it to track 300 households with patients in Liberia in the first week. More Than Me launched it shortly thereafter with awareness teams in West Point. "We have been using the app for contact tracing and with first responders," Sam Herring their data manager said. "Tomorrow we will begin capturing data on the needs of orphans and survivors."

The app's quick adoption is evidence that it does make work easier. The app was simple and stupid by design. The philosophy of a Lean Startup is to get something semi-functional into a user's hands immediately and build on what works. That way if nobody uses it, you've only wasted a few days and a few phones, rather than weeks of time designing the perfect solution for nobody. Facebook wasn't built "smart" on day one; it was a dumb hot-or-not picture sorting game launched in a dorm room in the wee hours of morning. And Ebola workers seem to be happy just to have some means of data coordination on the ground, even if it is buggy. The reason why More Than Me's ambulance picks up minutes instead of days later is because the system is simpler. There's one ambulance serving one local area and one specific person responsible. This app shares data about that previously isolated service with others.

The debate between JourneyApps and Chris Fabian of UNICEFstories.org illustrates one of the major rifts in how development works. Should we be lean and iterative or should we know what we are doing before we supply the complete solution?

Where both sides agree is that everything should be co-designed with the Africans that will use it. Too many past projects have been a waste because the people it was intended for were not involved in designing it. Fearing they were not involved in designing this app, Chris Fabian concluded, "I would rather dump the phones in the ocean than on west Africa."[5] The high rate of adoption by the intended users - local NGO workers - proves that they got something right.

The second and more intractable problem remains unsolved: People rarely consult data when making decisions.

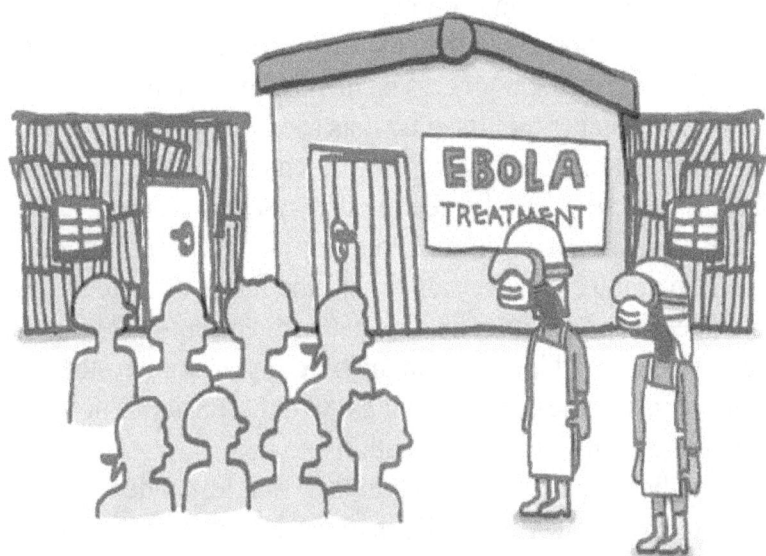

"Aid organizations need data to make decisions," the Ebola Care App's web page says[6]. This contains an unproven assumption. We want to believe that data automatically yields better decisions than no data, but all of my experience with leaders has shown that it doesn't matter. In governments and institutions alike, people make decisions based on their personal experience and wisdom first, then cite data to support the decision they *already made*. They are often unaware they think this way and will deny it. But it is the rare leader who weighs a decision solely on the evidence first, only later adding in a layer of personal experience. This is probably human nature, and unless we formally educate every citizen on how to think like a scientist or a judge, it will persist.

In our current system, people on the ground already make hundreds of decisions each day without looking at data. They may know past trends and the latest top-level statistics, like how many

Ebola cases there are in the country, but they don't examine the specific facts in real time, such as the life history of the next patient who walks through that door. Will they start using data if it becomes available? It depends. People often say they will, but if pouring over patterns costs them time they don't have, they won't.

The crux of the "app" problem is figuring out how to make the informed decision easier than the uninformed one. It's not enough for a decision-making process be merely better, it has to also be faster and cheaper too. Imagine if as soon as that person walks in for treatment, her life history was presented on screen with the top three risk factors for treatment. In this system a worker would have to consciously ignore information in front of him (i.e. opt out) to make an uninformed decision. That's the future of systems design, and I've written an essay about what such an "opt-out" system of democracy would look like on my blog if you're interested[7]. It works because the cost of making a wrong decision is now higher than the cost of finding information one needs.

Another organization trying to help first responders make decisions in West Africa is Keystone Accountability[8]. They just released their version of a lean solution - a weekly phone survey of 350 workers in the region about Ebola risks. They asked them to rate progress on several key areas that leaders in government and NGOs wanted to track. These are the questions, along with the average score for a recent poll[9] in parentheses after. On their 1 to 5 scale 1 means "not at all" and 5 means "very much so". I've sorted questions from highest to lowest scores to make the trends clearer:

Q2- Does fear of **stigmatisation** make people reluctant to report cases? (**4.2**)

Q8- Do **women and girls** have the same access to medical treatment as men? (**3.4**)

Q11- Overall, is the Ebola response **making progress** against the spread of the disease? (**3.1**)

Q7- Do people have **access to health care** if they get sick from non- Ebola diseases? (**2.6**)

Q9- Are the surveillance teams **responding to calls** quickly? **(2.4)**

Q10- Are people confident that if they call help lines, such as 117, their problems will be **dealt with promptly**? **(2.3)**

Q3- In your experience do people in quarantine have enough **food and water**? **(2.3)**

Q1- Do people follow **official quarantines** restrictions? **(2.1)**

Q5- Are the **burial teams** responding to calls quickly? **(2.1)**

Q6- Do you feel **safe and accepted** by people in the communities where you are working? **(2.0)**

Q4- Do people **trust the authorities** enough to do what they are told to prevent Ebola? **(1.9)**

Those with the lowest scores need immediate follow-up. People don't trust authorities and workers don't feel safe. Because of the way the question was worded, Q2 about stigma is also a huge problem, because it has the highest score (Stigma: "very much so!"). 70 percent of people were on the fence about whether we're making progress against the spread of disease (They answered 3 on a scale of 1 to 5). This is more optimistic than the mathematical projections, which still predict tens of thousands of cases by January 2015 in the "best case scenario." You have to wonder. If the lowest score went to peoples' trust of authorities, on what do they base their optimism that we are even holding steady against the spread of the disease? Local organizations and community leaders, I suspect.

This approach summarizes trends from a worker's perspective instead of a true bottom-up citizen's perspective. It's just that much harder to poll citizens, and so the results may even underestimate the severity of the problem. Keystone was thrilled to hear from me about Imani, More and Me, and other local organizations that were collecting statements from citizens about what they needed. They want to feed that into their summaries too, as what people ask for is a strong indicator on what parts of the problem remain unsolved.

While Keystone's results are easy for leaders to interpret and get updated on a weekly basis, what is less clear is whether the results will prompt action or just be used to justify what leaders were planning to do anyway. Perhaps the easier form of behavior change is to not focus on leaders, but rather, on citizens. Using technology to help the world's poor by giving them information has been a lofty, if unreachable goal for a long time now. Few have achieved transformational results. One essay by Ciara Byrne titled, "What I learned from building an app for low-income Americans" explains:[10]

> When doing nonprofit work it's all too easy to congratulate yourself for taking on the work at all. Technologists are problem solvers. It's tempting to either jump in too quickly with a technical solution to an intractable systemic or human problem or to be discouraged by its difficulty. One of my first interviews was with a 21-year-old father of two, Angel. Angel was in foster care before he turned one and had been in trouble with the law as a teenager. What he really needed was a steady job which would provide him with an income for his family. No mobile app I could build in three months was going to deliver that.

Poverty is a complex web of intractable problems. The author suggests solving the smallest part of a problem that you can instead of tackling everything:

> My colleague Jimmy Chen built a mobile app called EasyFoodStamps to do the first stage of the application for food stamps, saving people hours of standing in queues at the food stamp office. When you lose a day's work or have to get a babysitter to watch your kids in order to apply, that really makes a difference.

That food stamps app is a great example of a small but meaningful aid for the poor. My wife and I did an experiment and lived for 7 days on food stamps. It took us several hours just to calculate what our daily food stamp allowance would be in the District of Columbia. By the end we were hungry, malnourished, and getting sick, living on $2.67 a day.[11] Had we used this app, we might have qualified for more support.

In Africa the best example of mobile technology giving people income or saving them money has been M-PESA in Kenya. The concept was simple - anyone can send cash to anyone else in the form of an airtime voucher that can be converted into cash. By 2011, Kenyans were using M-PESA to transfer over a billion dollars to each other. The people who supposedly lived on $2 a day were sustaining a billion dollar mobile banking world. It went from zero to a billion in under three years[12]. Today and 40 percent of the country (17 million) is using it. This kind of success is unheard of.

But if the idea was simple and had massive demand, why was the SafariCom's M-PESA launch in Kenya the first one to really work? It had been tried over 60 times in other parts of Africa with only modest success. SafariCom figured out that something had been missing in other launches. Others had launched with 200 to 2000 places to cash out, primarily in rural areas. M-PESA started out with over 60,000 kiosks all over the country. Nobody was ever more than a few miles from a place where they could get cash. This was the difference.

Other attempts assumed that the primary use-case would be people in cities shopping with a phone account instead of a credit card, and so they only focuses on supporting users in cities. The unforeseen use-case was working people sending money back to the villages where their families lived within the same country. Previously, one of the kids would ride the bush taxi all day, cash in hand, to deliver it. Sometimes they'd get robbed, and frequently they'd miss school too. With M-PESA offering a pick up point even in small villages, families no longer had to provide their own courier service. As a bonus, school attendance increased too.

Building for the poor is often a guessing game. You don't get anywhere without the people you're trying to help taking a front seat in the design process. As Ciara Byrne explains further:[13]

Living on a low income translates into other forms of scarcity: of power, information, respect, opportunity, time, health, security, and even of sleep. Our job as app builders is to increase our users' stock of at least one of those resources.

Sometimes your potential users misunderstand or mistrust you. We had trouble persuading housecleaners and other domestic workers to come to interviews, even though we paid $25 per hour, which was higher than their regular hourly rate. They didn't know us and it looked too good to be true.

The most promising thing about this Ebola Care App isn't what it *can* do, but the number of Liberians and Sierra Leoneans that will be using it and defining what it *should* do. These are people who aren't used to being able to write the rules for themselves. The more they are in control, the easier Ebola will be to control. This app could give local organizations an advantage over the foreign billion dollar aid organizations, because now they can coordinate. And because behavior change is something that happens one relationship at a time, and local organizations are the ones with a wealth of relationships, they have greater "capacity."

Ciara Byrne offers one last anecdote:

A few years ago I interviewed a Mexican impact investor named Álvaro Rodríguez Arregui. He explained that impact investors need to be very clear about their motives. "Do you want to do good, or do you want to feel good?" he said. "It's much easier to feel good by giving away meals to starving kids in Sudan, but you are not going to solve any systemic problem in the world by doing that. In business you have to make hard decisions."

The hard decision here is not what to put in the app, but who to empower with the app. An app won't hold leaders accountable for not using the information that the app provides. Instead, local workers need to be making decisions with it. And like M-PESA, citizens need tools and information if they are going to contribute to their own well-being. Right now an army of health educators serve as the conduit of that knowledge, and that's the best we can do. But ultimately, top-down decision-making is a legacy system that is failing in the 21st century. Technology doesn't help one person see all the data and make a smarter decision. Instead, it helps every citizen see a little bit more information and make a smarter personal decision. The benefits propagate through society and big problems like health and corruption improve. This leads me to another sea-change in thinking about how we solve complex problems like Ebola. There is an approach to community behavior change that works at the individual level called "positive deviance." That's my next topic.

[1] https://chewychunks.wordpress.com/2013/07/02/4192/
[2] Go to http://0.facebook.com and you'll see the version of Facebook the other half sees.
[3] http://www.appsagainstebola.org/
[4] http://unicefstories.org/2014/11/17/dumping-smartphones-on-west-africa-is-a-bad-idea/
[5] http://unicefstories.org/2014/11/19/a-talk-with-apps-for-ebola-followup-to-dont-dump-phones-post/
[6] http://www.appsagainstebola.org/
[7] http://chewychunks.wordpress.com/2014/11/08/the-soul-of-justice-to-a-scientist-versus-a-lawyer/
[8] http://keystoneaccountability.org (In case you cared, I started consulting for them after writing this book.)
[9] Constituent Voice and the Ebola response. Ground Truth front line workers' survey: analysis of data Round One, November 21, 2014 - http://keystoneaccountability.wordpress.com/2014/11/18/would-you-recommend-this-ebola-response-to-a-friend/
[10] http://www.fastcolabs.com/3038792/what-i-learned-from-building-an-app-for-low-income-americans
[11] https://chewychunks.wordpress.com/2014/02/07/7-days-on-food-stamps-day-0-the-menu/
[12] http://www.safaricom.co.ke/mpesa_timeline/timeline.html
[13] http://www.fastcolabs.com/3038792/what-i-learned-from-building-an-app-for-low-income-americans

13: Positive deviants? Explain this behavior change thing once more to me!

In the reddit AMA we did in October of 2014, I answered 79 of the 200 questions on Ebola. The phrase I used more than any other - and the answer to how we stop it - was "behavior change."

Behavior change is hard. If it was easy we'd all be at the gym three days a week. Instead we're in line for a burger that often.

The traditional, middle ages way of forcing behavior change is coercion. "Attend our church or we'll throw you in prison!" was a pretty common attitude back then. The same penalties are still imposed for engaging in controversial social behaviors around the world today. Sierra Leone made it a crime to hide an Ebola patient[1]. And traditional healers and churches in Liberia were prosecuted for their behavior on similar grounds[2]. Uganda famously criminalized being gay. None of these laws changed behavior because coercion is a pretty weak incentive. If a person really wants to do it, they're going to do it, and no amount of policing will stop it.

The opposite of coercion is positive deviance[3]. The concept is easier to illustrate through the story of how it started[4] than to describe.

In 1991, Communist Vietnam didn't want any foreign organizations meddling with their country. At the same time, they ranked very low on the global health index and needed to demonstrate that they were improving lives. Save the Children had been lobbying the government to be let in, and reluctantly officials agreed.

"You have six months to show improvements," they were told. "If you fail, you're out again."

A married couple - the Sternins - were invited in and told to create an effective child malnutrition program. Two thirds of village children were malnourished at the time. The government knew that giving them bags of rice had no lasting effect after the supplements ended. And the short time frame eliminated copying anything Save the Children had ever done before.

The Sternins came up with a radically different approach. They did what made sense. In four villages with 2,000 children they invited the community to identify poor families who had managed to avoid malnutrition. These neighbors faced the same obstacles as everyone else, but somehow were better off.

They started a dialogue. Highlighting the people the villagers chose and role models, they asked, "What do you know about this family that is different from you?"

They brainstormed, offered ideas, and debated. Someone took notes. Then they brought up the next family.

By the end of the meeting they had a chalk board full of things that some people were doing in the community that the others were not previously thinking about. Then the Sternins asked them to discuss and agree upon one specific thing from the list of better-off families that everyone would try for the next month. This was the "intervention" that would be applied to the village. No external authority, no peer-reviewed literature, and no randomized controlled trial informed the decision. Only a community's consensus, shared desire, and neighbor's success did.

One community chose to emulate a family that collected tiny shrimps and crabs from paddy fields, and added those, along with sweet potato greens, to their children's meals. The villagers had thought they were inappropriate to feed to young children before, but now were willing to give it a try. "If it's good enough for Phuong's baby, it's good enough for my kids."

Another village realized that the role-model mothers were feeding their children three to four times a day, instead of just twice, as was customary.

In a third village mothers of well-nourished kids had very strict hygiene. Children would always wash their hands before eating, and what-do-you-know, they're not sick as much, so they gain weight faster.

Through these community inquiry meetings, community members had discovered for themselves what it took for a very poor family to have a well-nourished child. But witnessing this discrepancy in health was not the behavior change mechanism alone. They also needed to practice it.

The magic of the positive deviance approach can be wrapped up inside this one koan:

"It is easier to act your way into a new way of thinking, than to think your way into a new way of acting."

It actually came from a Thanh Hoa saying, "Mot ghin nghe, khong bang mot xem, mot xem khong bank mot ghin lam" - which means:

"a thousand hearings isn't worth one seeing, and a thousand seeings isn't worth one doing."

In this spirit, the Sternins decided not to charge anybody with the task of "spreading the word." Instead, they brought mothers and their malnourished children to a neighbor's house for a few hours every day where someone who already had good habits would help the newbie do the new practice. It might seem so simple - just go out in the rice paddy and get shrimp and put it in a bowl - but it is the act of sharing the chore with a friend that makes it stick.

Every day, each mother or caretaker was required to bring a handful of shrimps, crabs or greens as the price of admission to the sessions. For two weeks every month, someone in the family, (a spouse, an older sibling), had to go out to the rice paddy early in the morning, and ankle deep in the mud, collect the required shrimps and crabs. By the fifteenth morning, the daily trip to the rice paddy with a small net and empty tin can had become routine and was continued.

This is behavior change. The knowledge of what one ought to do is easy to transfer, but the pattern of one's life only changes when the intervention interrupts a schedule in exactly this way.

Over six months the community discovered together what worked, and permanently changed their daily habits. These role models were known as "positive" because they were doing things right, and "deviants" because they engaged in behaviors that most others did not. The project showed dramatic improvements in child nutrition and the team was allowed to continue.

That's where the official narrative[5] leaves off, but not where the story ends. In the process of finding what works, each village had solved the problem in a different way. The local success were great for them, but offered no solution that could be copied elsewhere, critics said. Even within Save the Children Federation itself, such an approach put teams of experts and evaluators and randomized-controlled-trialers out of work. The battle between the randomistas ("one solution to rule them all") and the complexicons ("each island its own paradise") rages on to this day. In our search for universal solutions, we've left behind many of the most effective solutions, because those only work in the specific village where they were tested. The Sternins noted that another village just a few kilometers away from the first one couldn't add shrimp to their kids' food, because it wasn't available.

The only way this approach works across many contexts is to give each person who needs to change the means to see the world as it is, then let her decide what she will change in her own life. Then, after she tries it, we help her understand if she is better off. This process is exactly where we arrived in the last chapter about smart phone apps and decision-making. Positive deviance is simply a way to convert the information that apps provide into muscle memory. Without it, knowledge has no impact. It doesn't change lives.

Many of the successes in this book in stopping Ebola are examples of behavior change. Women stopped touching corpses when mourning for the dead, ending a tradition that goes as far back as written history. Friends now shake elbows instead of hands when they meet. Customers wash their hands in chlorine water when entering and exiting shops. Police take temperatures instead of bribes (We wish! I'm sure bribery is still a frequent part of their daily habits, sadly.) And people are starting to report the sick and the dying to hotlines so that others will come pick up the bodies. Trust in government remains at an all-time low. It is another one of these "intractable" problems, one that only positive deviance could be powerful enough to solve. Ebola was able to easily spread in West Africa because government leaders there had exploited the poor and powerless for decades, destroying any trust in government. When an existential threat appeared, nobody was willing to believe the government nor comply with rules. It should give you pause that today, fewer American citizens trust their government than at any point in recent history[6]. We need a government that is worthy of trust and citizens willing to trust it, but neither side is going to budge without some sort of "kick start." Positive deviance would have government leaders who are more trusted and competent than the rest be the role models for the most corrupt ones. The crooks and the do-nothings would be forced to shadow the a role model around for weeks at a time, doing exactly what he/she does, practicing the new behaviors, until such habits are ingrained. Most of the time incompetence is a function of the system, and borrowing "good" bureaucrats across agencies and systems would quickly reveal where the system is the problem, and any person in that role is guaranteed to stink. This isn't an easy thing to fix, and nearly impossible without experimentation. We have to "act our way into a new way of thinking" if we want to be a resilient society.

---

[1] http://www.voanews.com/content/sierra-leone-criminalizes-hiding-ebola-patients/2425906.html
[2] http://www.smh.com.au/world/ebola-toll-jumps-to-467-worst-outbreak-on-record-20140701-zssri.html
[3] http://www.positivedeviance.org/
[4] http://www.positivedeviance.org/about_pd/Monique%20VIET%20NAM%20CHAPTER%20Oct%2017.pdf
[5] http://www.positivedeviance.org/
[6] http://www.gallup.com/poll/5392/trust-government.aspx

14: What can I do to help? Empathize, don't sympathize.

Empathy is a mirroring of human emotions. Empathy is stepping into someone else's world, rather than looking at it from over the fence. It is different from sympathy, which is when you acknowledge someone else's pain and comfort them, but keep the experience at arm's length. Empathy is about embracing the struggle and injecting yourself into the experience. There is an RSAanimate video of philosophy Roman Krznaric explains why only empathy makes the world a better place[1]. I've shared screen-shots of a few key points here.

"We need to shift from introspection to outrospection," Roman says. "Discover the lives of other people and other civilizations." Take for example, Che Guevara. He became a revolutionary leader after exploring his continent and being shocked at the poverty and powerlessness.

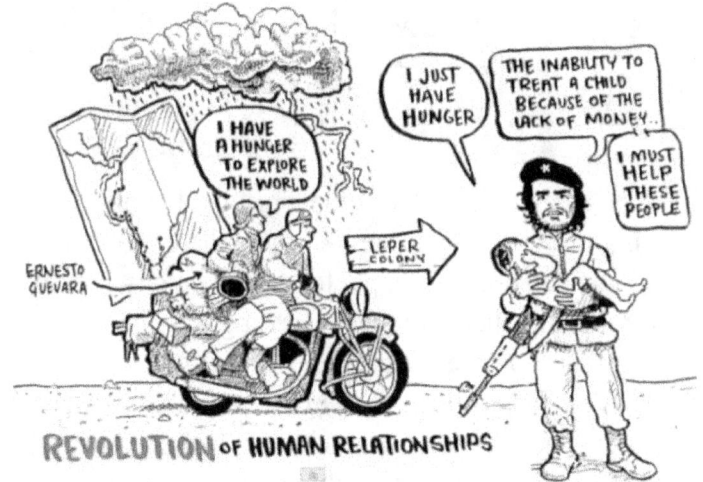

"We have prejudices about other people which block us from seeing them," Roman says, "and highly empathetic people get beyond labels by nurturing their curiosity for others. Empathy brings about a revolution in human relationships."

And how do we nature this kind of curiosity? Roman proposes a different kind of museum - an empathy museum.

the empathy museum

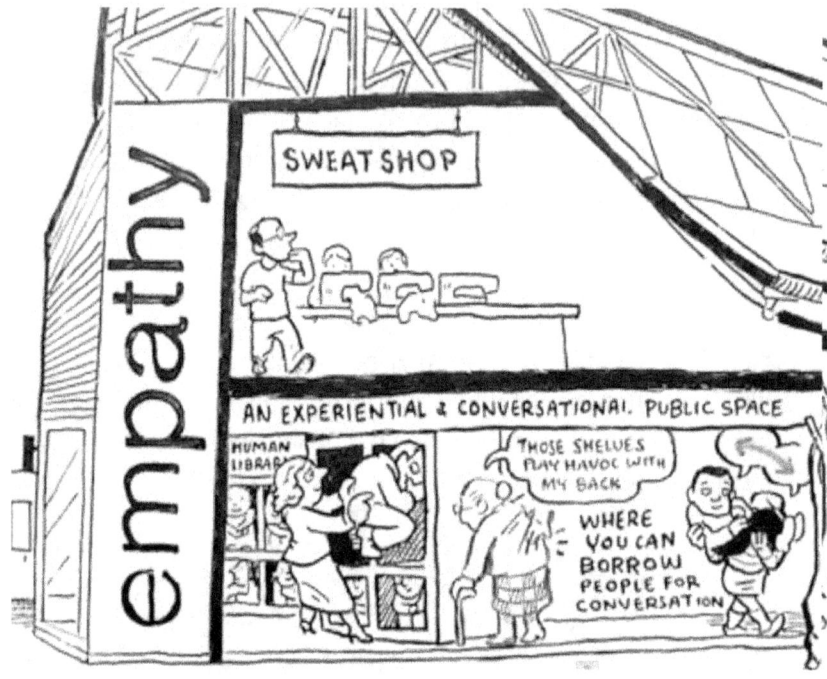

"It would be an experiential and conversational public space, where you might walk in and in the first room there is a human library where you can borrow people for conversations. You walk into the next room and there are twenty sewing machines. And there are former Vietnamese sweat shop workers who will teach you how to make a T-shirt like the one you are probably wearing under sweatshop labour conditions, and you'll be paid 5 pence at the end of it, so you understand the labour behind the labels….

I think we need to think about brining empathy into our every day lives in a very habitual way."

These two elements - conversations and habits - are deeply ingrained with our identity and circle of friends. We habitually converse with the people we're closest to. It is an unfortunate side-effect of technology that many of us live our lives surrounded almost entirely by people who see the world as we want to see it, and don't necessarily see the world for what it is. The few that bridge different worlds tend to be better traveled, and infrequent consumers of television, games, and other catered content. You've probably heard that highly processed food has less nutrition? I believe highly processed content is also missing a certain emotional-spiritual rawness that all humans need in order to blossom as empathizers. You can flip a channel or switch websites or buy a different game, but you can't shut a person up who is telling you some uncomfortable fact about the world. It helps when you've seen part of the world yourself, and you can judge what this person has to say from some realistic frame of reference. Recently I was very happy when I saw the transformation of an idea about what counter-terrorism operations meant. From this:

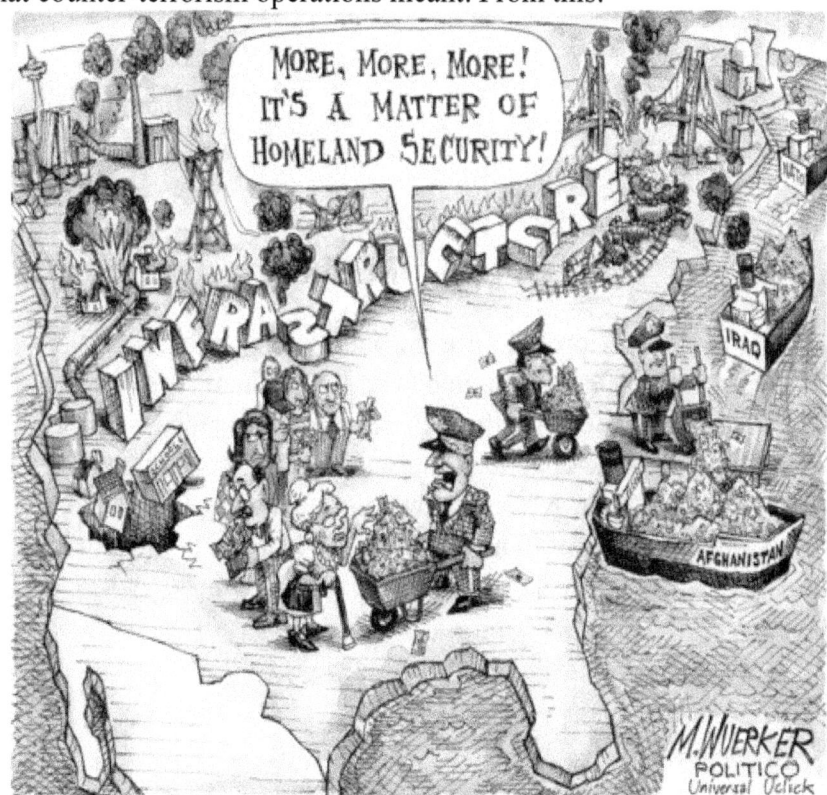

To this:

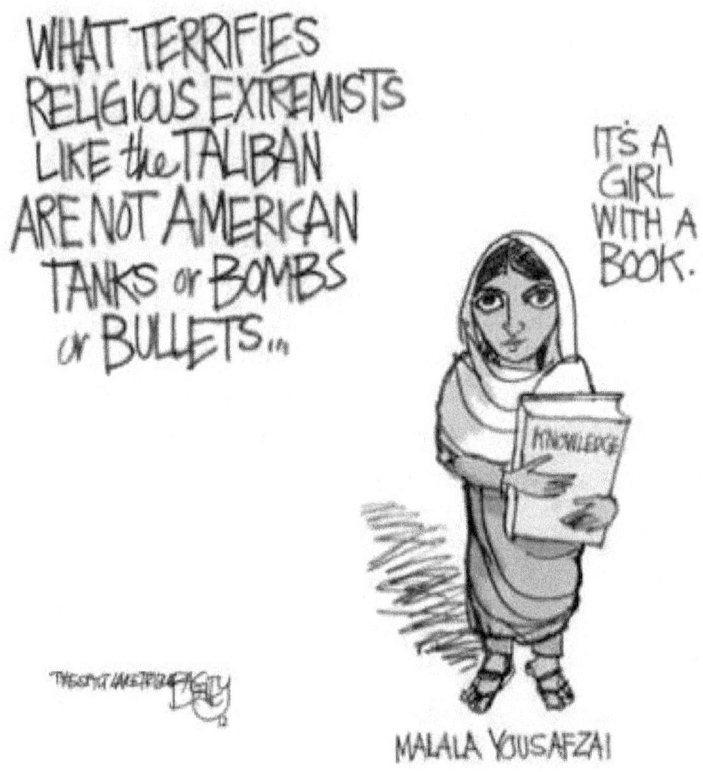

WHAT TERRIFIES RELIGIOUS EXTREMISTS LIKE the TALIBAN ARE NOT AMERICAN TANKS or BOMBS or BULLETS...

IT'S A GIRL WITH A BOOK.

KNOWLEDGE

MALALA YOUSAFZAI

I made an effort to infuse raw local voices into this book, because people are better able to speak for themselves than any of us are able to speak for them. A diversity of perspectives is healthy, even therapeutic, because it leads to more empathy.

The shift from sympathy towards empathy has started to make its way into popular thought. The last five years of Google internet searches show that "empathy" is replacing "sympathy"[2]:

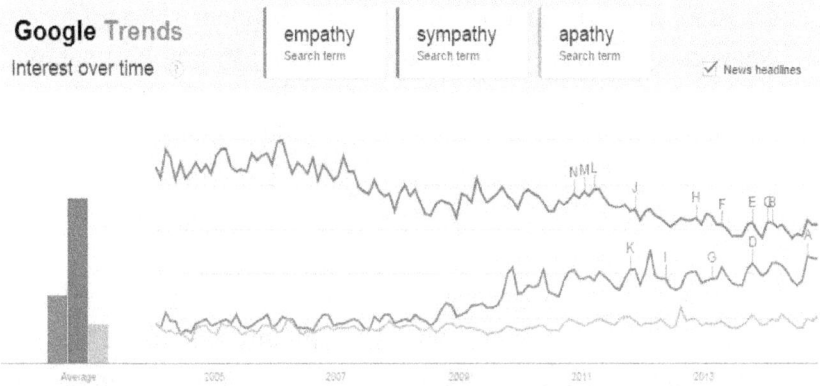

It's a hopeful trend that people are thinking more about this, but what specific actions could you take right now that would matter?

The history of social change (slavery, human rights, racism, etc.) is really the story of the rise and fall of empathy within populations. So if you want a safer world, go start a conversation with someone nothing like yourself. Just one coffee date with your nemesis could change the world. And if it doesn't change the world, at least you've changed the world within your reach.

There are probably better ways to find your anti-self, but this is how I would do it. Sign up on Okcupid.com and create a profile. When they ask you what you are looking for, select **"For new friends"** instead of the usual romantic options. Then answer a few questions about yourself to train their matching algorithm. Go to "Browse matches" and order your search results by **"Enemy %"**:

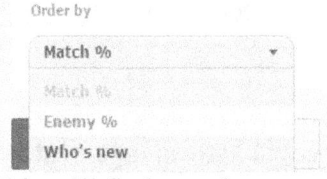

This will find you the person you have the most to learn from of all the people in your town or city. Email them and invite them out for coffee.

I just tried it. My 99% enemy for the Washington, DC area is a 21 year old girl with two kids who says she "is emo, listens to screamo, and been arrested 6 times." The statement "my favorite weapon is nife" also makes it into the first paragraph somehow. And she's passionate about "beating up dweebs."

It's going to be really, really interesting meeting my nemesis. Oh the things I do for science![3] [Update: I am not legally responsible for whatever happens on your nemesis date. Just sayin'.]

If the thought of starting a dialogue scares you, you can always go to www.globalgiving.org/ebola right now and give $100 to support dozens of local organizations working around the clock to stop Ebola in West Africa. They'll be happy to go out into the community and start life-saving dialogues with your money. As a bonus, you'll get regular email updates from all the organizations working there.

Epilogue

Putting it back in context of my original premise - how we react to a crisis defines what kind of person we are - we have a moral obligation to listen. Are we the victims of someone else's fear mongering, or are we looking for facts, listening to the people on the ground, and gathering their perspective? Do we put ourselves in their shoes (empathy) and make decisions that would help them? I hope these stories have given you a better understanding of what Ebola is really like, and how our choices build up or break down systems that could save us from ourselves. Even leaders need our empathy too, because we are all interconnected now.

Acknowledgements

Without the hard work of many people in local organizations in Liberia, Sierra Leone, Guinea, and elsewhere, there would be nothing to write about. They deserve the biggest thanks for their tireless, thankless, gruelling efforts. In particular, Katie, Emily, and M. Holden Warren (photographer) of More Than Me contributed. I also appreciate the team at the GlobalGiving Foundation, especially Britt, Will, and Alison who invited me into the Reddit AMA that launched many of these questions. And lastly, a big thank you to Christy my wife for putting up with the 50 hours of research over 6 weeks it took to find good source material. The work is never done, but I hope this installment bring you - the reader - a little closer to the reality on the ground.

---

[1] https://www.youtube.com/watch?v=BG46IwVfSu8
[2] https://chewychunks.wordpress.com/2013/01/09/empathy-replaces-sympathy-rsa-animate/
[3] https://chewychunks.wordpress.com/2012/12/19/marcs-dating-dashboard-tracking-impact-in-international-development/

Appendix

How do people get Ebola?

The level of risk is defined below based on CDC recommendations [20].

High risk - A high-risk exposure includes any of the following:
- Percutaneous (e.g., needle stick) or mucous membrane exposure to blood or body fluids (e.g., feces, saliva, sweat, urine, vomit, and semen) of a person with symptomatic Ebola virus disease
- Exposure to the blood or body fluids (e.g., feces, saliva, sweat, urine, vomit, and semen) of a person with symptomatic Ebola virus disease without appropriate personal protective equipment (PPE)
- Processing blood or other body fluids of a person with symptomatic Ebola virus disease without appropriate PPE or standard biosafety precautions
- Direct contact with a dead body without appropriate PPE in a country with widespread Ebola virus transmission
- Having lived in the immediate household and provided direct care to a person with symptomatic Ebola virus disease

Some risk - Some risk of exposure includes any of the following:
- In countries with widespread Ebola virus transmission: direct contact while using appropriate PPE with a person with symptomatic Ebola virus disease
- Close contact in households, healthcare facilities, or community settings with a person with Ebola while the person was symptomatic. Close contact is defined as being within approximately three feet (one meter) of the infected person for a prolonged period of time while not wearing appropriate PPE

Low risk - A low-risk exposure includes any of the following:

• Having been in a country with widespread Ebola virus transmission within the past 21 days, but without any known exposures to Ebola virus

• Having brief direct contact (e.g., shaking hands) while not wearing appropriate PPE, with a person with Ebola while the person was in the early stage of disease

• Brief proximity, such as being in the same room for a brief period of time, with a person with symptomatic Ebola virus disease

• In countries without widespread Ebola virus transmission: direct contact while using appropriate PPE with a person with symptomatic Ebola virus disease

• Travel on an aircraft with a person with symptomatic Ebola virus disease, without direct physical contact

No identifiable risk - Some exposures or situations have no identifiable risk of infection. These include:

• Contact with an asymptomatic person who had contact with a person with Ebola

• Contact with a person who is later diagnosed with Ebola virus disease, before the person developed symptoms

• Having been in a country with widespread Ebola virus transmission more than 21 days previously

• Having been in a country without widespread Ebola virus transmission and not having any other exposures as defined above

These guidelines have been used to identify at-risk individuals during the 2014 outbreak in West Africa. Individuals may also be at risk for Ebola disease if they have handled bats, rodents, or non-human primates from other endemic areas of Africa.[1]

Where can I follow the story of the 2014-2015 Ebola outbreak?

By the numbers: The *New York Times* has an excellent resource that they update weekly from other primary reports (MSF, WHO, CDC, etc) at http://www.nytimes.com/interactive/2014/07/31/world/africa/ebola-virus-outbreak-qa.html. This is just one of dozens of interactive charts:

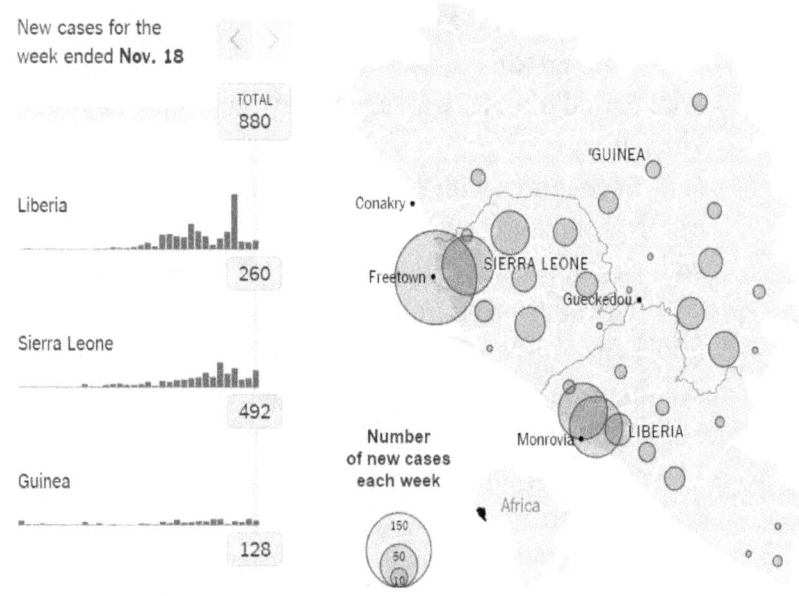

Interesting to note the giant spike in Liberian cases a few weeks before Nov 18th. That was the result of auditing old records and updating them. The size of the spike is an indication of how much the outbreak has been undercounting cases due to a lack of manpower.

Follow Katie Meyler of More Than Me in Liberia on her tumblr page: http://RacingHeartBlog.tumblr.com

www.eboladeeply.com offers a good digest of local voices.

I re-blog stories told by the people directly affected on my blog: http://ebolastories.wordpress.com

Thanks for reading! I would love to hear your feedback.

Marc Maxmeister

---

[1] http://www.uptodate.com/contents/diagnosis-and-treatment-of-ebola-and-marburg-virus-disease?source=see_link

www.ingramcontent.com/pod-product-compliance
Lightning Source LLC
Chambersburg PA
CBHW051811170526
45167CB00005B/1963